CRYSTAL RX

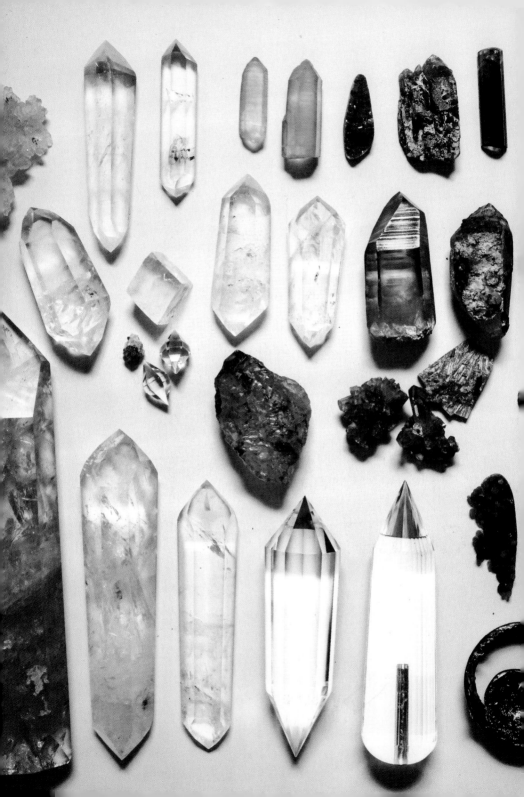

CRYSTAL RX

Daily Rituals for Cultivating Calm,
Achieving Your Goals, and Rocking
Your Inner Gem Boss

COLLEEN McCANN

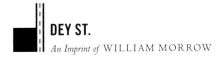

DEY ST.
An Imprint of WILLIAM MORROW

DEY ST.

CRYSTAL RX. Copyright © 2018 by Colleen McCann. All rights reserved. Printed in the United States of America. No part of this book may be used or reproduced in any manner whatsoever without written permission except in the case of brief quotations embodied in critical articles and reviews. For information, address HarperCollins Publishers, 195 Broadway, New York, NY 10007.

HarperCollins books may be purchased for educational, business, or sales promotional use. For information, please e-mail the Special Markets Department at SPsales@harpercollins.com.

FIRST EDITION

Designed by Michelle Crowe

Library of Congress Cataloging-in-Publication Data has been applied for.

ISBN 978-0-06-284444-6

18 19 20 21 22 LSC 10 9 8 7 6 5 4 3 2 1

May you walk in beauty always and forever. *Aho!*

"Walk in beauty" is a Navajo blessing and prayer similar in meaning to "state of grace" in Christianity or *shalom* in Hebrew. When one is walking in beauty, one is in harmony with everything around them, recognizing the beauty and interconnectedness of everything encountered in a heightened state of awareness. I am honored to teach "the beauty way" in more ways than one. In various native languages, *aho* translates to hello, thank you, amen, good-bye, and, as I like to look at it, "Yeah, babe, I hear what you're saying, and I like it."

CONTENTS

Introduction   1

1 — Crystals 101: An Intro to Stone Medicine   11

2 — Building Your Crystal Arsenal   59

3 — Crystal Intelligence:
What Does Science Have to Say?   93

4 — Your Mini Encyclopedia of Crystals   109

5 —— Rock It! Crystals in Every Area of Your Life 145

6 —— Crystals and the Zodiac 213

7 —— Let's Go Exploring 229

The Crystal Life 257

Acknowledgments 259

Credits 263

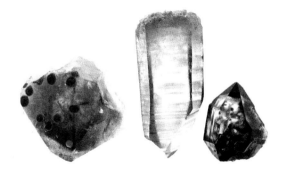

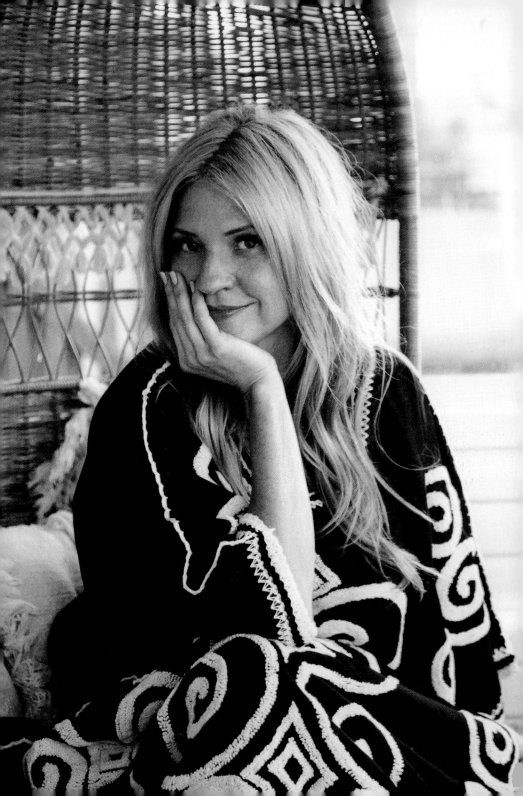

INTRODUCTION

The [wo]man who moves a mountain begins by
carrying away small stones.

–CONFUCIUS

HI, I'M COLLEEN, and I'm a shaman—though I'm probably not your typical shaman (I also happen to wear fake eyelashes and high heels to work). I spend my days conducting intuitive crystal readings with clients, teaching Shaman School, working with the editorial community on mystically minded content, and talking at speaking engagements about my favorite thing—crystals! But it wasn't always this way. In my "past life," I was a fashion stylist, which I did successfully for fifteen years, living your typical life in New York City. Then, ten years ago I got a personal ping from the universe telling me it was time to make a huge life shift. I started having premonitions, seeing spirits/apparitions, hearing voices, and being told by complete strangers on the street that I was a healer. *What was happening?*

Before I answer that, let's backtrack a bit. I grew up your typical Midwestern Irish Catholic girl, but there were signs all along, from the moment I entered this world, that I was meant to embrace the mystical life. I was born in Pittsburgh, Pennsylvania, on the day of the High Priestess (August 29, making me a Virgo, the sign of the Healer), during an intense electrical storm. My mom had a contraction every time lightning streaked or thunder crashed outside the hospital window. Years later, an astrologer would explain to me that this was a very auspicious weather pattern, due to the specific alignment of the planets at the time of my birth.

As a kid, I always had an uncanny intuitive sense. At age seven, I woke up one morning and somehow just knew the winning numbers to that night's pick-3 lotto jackpot. I convinced my mom to buy a ticket, and the $2,000 prize money allowed my family to buy a totally boss camcorder. I also stunned my first-grade teacher, Sister Mathias, by guessing the *exact* number of gumballs in the glass jar in our classroom. This ability, known as *claircognizance*—when someone *just knows*, though they can't explain why or how they got the information—started for me when I was small. I still have it today, though now I work with my intuition in a professional setting, relying on my skills to conduct Intuitive Crystal Readings, Psychic Business Building Sessions, or Shamanic Closet Cleansings for my clients.

MY SPIRITUAL JOURNEY

Crystals have long been a part of my life, though it took me some time to realize that they were my calling. I have always been drawn to blingy statement jewelry, but it wasn't until I set foot in my first metaphysical shop eleven years ago, on the random recommendation of a friend, that I began to discover the real power of gemstones. A metaphysical shop or "New Age" store is one that houses tools and educational materials—like tarot cards, books, candles, sage, pendulums, and, of course, crystals—related to spiritual or religious beliefs and practices.

The moment I walked into this shop, I locked eyes with a woman named SheyShey (which means "thank you" in Chinese) who would completely change my life and end up becoming my first crystals mentor. But at the time, I was a skeptic. "What can I help you find?" SheyShey asked as she approached me. My sarcastic inner voice was screaming, *My sanity!* but all I managed to say was, "I don't know." SheyShey replied, "Well, look around and see what speaks to you." I started browsing the shelves and chose several crystal necklaces based on their radiant color and intricate textures. SheyShey looked at me and said, "Oh, you aren't happy with some of the relationships in your life. I don't think you are happy in your career, and you want to make more money. Plus, you are feeling lost and looking for clarity." I was stunned, and found myself holding back tears, as everything she had just said was correct. "How did you know those things?" I asked. She smiled mysteriously and said, "By the crystals you chose, of course. Each crystal has a certain meaning. We wear crystals to help us with what we are trying to work on in life." How was her intuition so spot-on? I walked out of the store trying to make sense of what had just happened—and with three necklaces: Rose Quartz for love, Clear Quartz for clarity, and Citrine for abundance in business (SheyShey had explained their meaning to me). That night, lying in bed with my new purchases around my neck, I replayed the day's events in my head, my mind racing. I had to know more!

I went back to see SheyShey a few weeks later. She greeted me warmly and asked, "What stones are speaking to you today?" I picked up two more necklaces, and she immediately said "Oh, you are having trouble with your voice. You have many important things to tell him, but you are holding back. You are also about to start traveling more for work, so those are a good choice, too." Again, I stared at her, wide-eyed. There was indeed someone in my life who I needed to have a heart-to-heart with, I just didn't have the balls to do it. I had also just signed on for an ongoing project that paid well—and that would put me on airplanes about 75 percent of the time. I told her this. Her response? "Oh, good, the Citrine is working nicely for you." (This amazing job had material-ized *after* my first visit to the store, when I'd bought the Citrine necklace for business abundance.) I bought the two new necklaces without hesi-tation this time, thus adding Lapis Lazuli, stone of communication, and Tiger's Eye, stone of protection in travel, to my arsenal.

SheyShey had blown my mind, and I went back to see her again and again, to learn from her and to build my collection. Eventually I became a permanent fixture in the store, where I would sit on a little wooden bench and listen (which felt reminiscent of sitting in a church pew every Sunday through my childhood), absorbing everything that SheyShey had to teach me like a sponge. I learned that SheyShey was Chinese, a Buddhist, and a lawyer turned "Crystals Master," and she has since become one of my greatest teachers. I am eternally grateful that she was so patient with me that first day in the shop, and that she took me under her wing and gave me my start in the world of crystals. Everything that I am about to share with you, I owe to her.

Not long after first meeting SheyShey, some strange things began to happen. I like to think of them as signs from the universe that my life, and my calling, was about to change. I heard my first "voice," also known as *clairaudience*—in a Brooklyn bodega, of all places, predicting that another customer and the cashier were going to get into a fight over the price of bananas. A few days later, I was walking through Midtown Manhattan, about to cross Fifth Avenue, when I heard the same voice from the bodega say, "*Stop, stop, stop—go left!"* Instead of crossing the street, I stopped dead in my tracks at the corner, and I watched the man who'd been walking next to me on my left side get clipped by a car on his right. Fortunately, he wasn't hurt, but I would have been a goner had I kept walking! Several similarly eerie and prophetic events followed, including a psychic-medium woman at Mercedes-Benz Fashion Week who wanted to examine my vibrant green aura. I also started to notice, quite frequently, that when my iPhone was facedown and would ding, I knew exactly who it was without looking. I wrote this off at first, but then it happened with someone I hadn't heard from or seen in over five years. *Okay, Universe, I hear you loud and clear.*

My next stop was a consultation with reputable New York City–based psychic and healer Asa Hoffman, who took one look at me and said, "Honey, you're not crazy, you're psychic!" He explained over the course of our session that the voices were in fact my "Spirit Guides" saying hello. The premonitions were my clairvoyance, also called "second sight," kicking in, which means I'm able to perceive things or events from the past or in the future that are beyond normal sensory observation. Premonitions come to me in the form of movielike images, both when I'm awake and dreaming. Asa told me I needed to get a spiritual mentor, pronto, because my whole life was about to change.

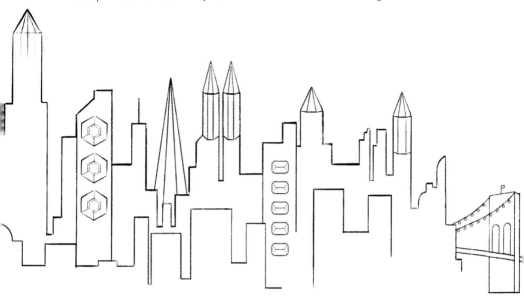

COMING OUT OF THE
SHAMANIC CLOSET

As I continued my trip down the crystal-laden rabbit hole, it became clear on many levels that my career as a fashion stylist was no longer the great-fitting LBD it once had been. I began to feel like I was leading a double life—no one else knew that I was splitting my time between shamanic studies and the fashion world. I started to feel a lot of internal conflict. There were still so many things I loved about the fashion world—collaborating with creative types to build a collective vision on a project and watching it come to life before my eyes, the magnetic energy on set, traveling to exotic locations, freedom of expression, and of course the endless visual array of patterns, colors, and textures of the designer clothing—but on set, it became impossible to ignore the industry's toxic side (greed, vanity, ego, addiction, and workaholicism, with a whopping side of eating disorders). Not to mention that being a fashion stylist is backbreaking work, involving long hours and perpetual jetlag. Something had to change.

Interestingly, as my spiritual knowledge increased, I seemed to become a magnet for those seeking counsel. I'd be backstage with a gaggle of naked Glamazons, and out of nowhere one would start spilling her emotional and spiritual guts to me, asking for my advice. I'd stand there, a sacred witness, being cried on and hugged by a statuesque beauty with her tits in my face (literally, because I'm five foot two). After several of these mildly uncomfortable moments, I decided to put my training to work and began sharing the ancient wisdom teachings that I was learning— with my own uniquely curated spin. I would give each of these ladies "mystical homework," and a "Crystal Rx" for what ailed them. Imagine my surprise when I started getting their follow-up emails thanking me for my advice and telling me how much it was helping. *Was I onto something?*

As a stylist, I traveled constantly—from the runways of Paris to the crystal caves of South America—and on these journeys, I began to merge my two great loves: fashion and mysticism. As I became more and more spiritually attuned, I began to incorporate my healing knowledge with everyone I encountered, from models backstage to strangers in airports. And this is how Style Rituals was born. I'd always had a deep appreciation for all things beautiful and been acutely aware of the power and strength that lies in the exquisite. But I also believe that there is power in beauty only when beauty exudes honesty, strength, compassion, and confidence. This realization is what catapulted me into merging my two passions into one unique vision, and it became the underlying philosophy behind my business.

Of course, launching Style Rituals took time (two months locked in my bedroom developing a business plan and a website) and plenty of effort. I had to get my fashionista clientele on board with the idea of booking crystal healing sessions with a prophetess who had formerly chosen their outfits and curated their closets. But little by little, and as people started to see results, my client list grew through word of mouth. Because crystal healing is for real, and I was bringing it to my clients in a way that didn't feel too woo-woo or New Age. Some ingredients in my secret sauce included prescribing crystal

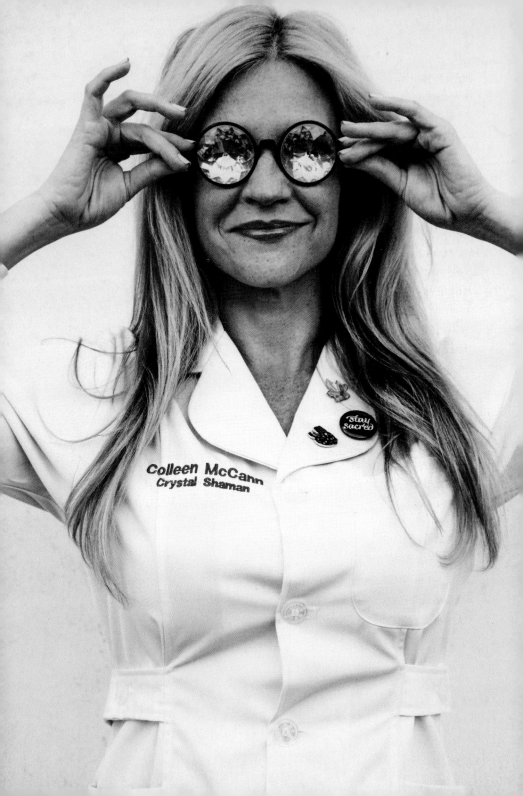

prescriptions with palatable and memorable nicknames that my well-dressed community could relate to. I'd compare different crystal usages to clothing, self-care rituals, Xanax and Botox during my signature Intuitive Crystal Reading (a custom blend of techniques from many different healing modalities wrapped into a one-hour sesh), plus my Chakra Cleanse, which I describe as "a green juice detox for the soul" (more on these later!).

My goal in this book is to do the same thing for you that I do for each of my private clients in our sessions. I want to teach you the ancient art of Stone Medicine, updated for the twenty-first century and tailored to your needs! As you will learn in this book, there is a Crystal Rx for just about everything. Through working with stones and crystals, we can heal mentally, physically, emotionally, and spiritually. Crystals can help us to increase focus and clarity, silence anxiety and depression, curb addictions, build confidence, improve our communication skills, make better life choices, heal relationship traumas, and even get sounder sleep. All we need is the know-how.

So follow me into the wilds of the crystal kingdom. On our journey, you will meet thought leaders from various industries who are finding fascinating new ways to use crystals in both their business and personal practices. I want the world to understand how palatable Crystal Medicine is, and how crystals can be incorporated in so many areas of life, from beauty to fashion to music to technology to food. Crystals are becoming big business, attracting followers who range from celebrities to Wall Street bankers to Hollywood screenwriters to real estate titans. I'll also share plenty of tips, tricks, and how-tos along the way to help you develop your own personal practice and curate your crystal collection. The world of crystals is changing at lightning speed—no longer hippie-dippie, it's an increasingly sophisticated and growing industry.

Let's go!

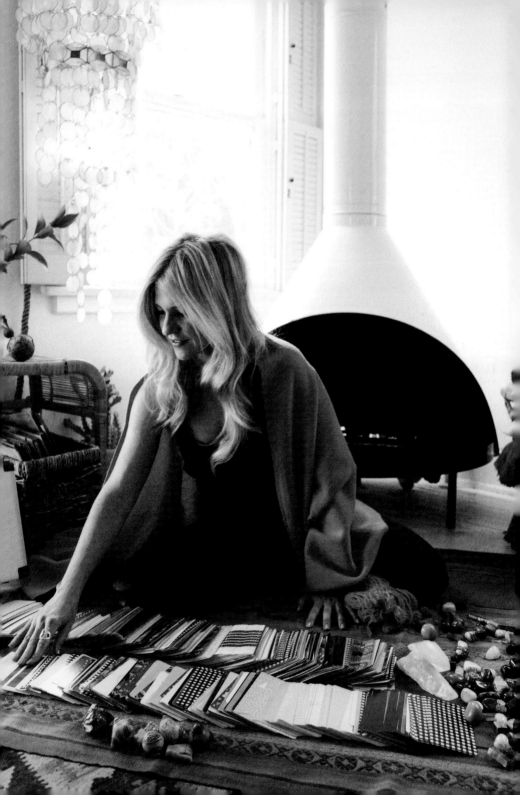

1

CRYSTALS 101

An Intro to Stone Medicine

Throw your dreams into space like a kite, and you do not
know what it will bring back, a new life, a new friend,
a new love, a new country.

—ANAÏS NIN

WE OFTEN HEAR CRYSTALS REFERRED TO AS "NEW AGE," but
in truth, crystal healing is an ancient, age-old form of medicine. Crystal
healing is woven into the threads of some of our most historic civiliza-
tions. The Mayas, Incas, ancient Egyptians, Australian Aborigines, Native Americans, Celtic Druids, and more all traditionally used crystals in
their healing practices. Shamans refer to the practice of placing crystals
on someone's body for healing purposes as "the laying on of stones."

Crystal healing is a holistic, noninvasive, vibrationally based system
of energetic healing. Sparkly crystals, river rocks, polished stones, or
faceted gems are laid at precise locations on and/or around a person's
body to facilitate healing. Crystal healers believe that this practice
treats the physical body as well as the LEF (Luminous Energy Field)

around the body (also known as the Auric Body, the Auric Field, or the Energy Field). As crystals interact with people and the physical and energetic space surrounding us, they can absorb, defuse, direct, detoxify, focus, and shift our energy.

WHAT IS BEING "HEALED," EXACTLY?

In this context, "healing" means bringing balance to the mind, body, spirit, and physical space. Shamans believe that everything starts on an energetic level and then manifests mentally, physically, or emotionally. Negative energy, or "dis-ease," can show itself through physical illnesses and behavioral issues, which are the final manifestation of ancestral, emotional, environmental, karmic, mental, physiological, psychological, or spiritual imbalances. Crystal healing helps restore the body to its natural equilibrium, but keep in mind that it's meant to be an accoutrement to other health treatments. Always consult a healthcare professional on what your personal path should be, and how you can combine Eastern and Western medicine for best results.

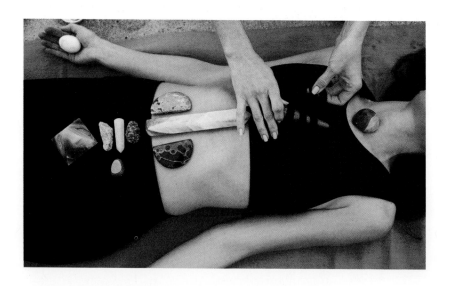

WHAT DO PEOPLE EXPERIENCE DURING CRYSTAL HEALING?

Most commonly I hear clients say, "I feel better, even if I can't pinpoint why." The process is very therapeutic and relaxing, and it creates a safe space to release unwanted energy; people may laugh, cry, or fall asleep. They can feel very energized, euphoric, or extremely tired after a session. Some people may sense "a presence in the room," or feel something touch their arm. People sometimes get visions or bursts of creative ideas. Some experience a sensation of floating or leaving their body, which in the biz is called "astral projection." There are also muscle jerks or tingling sensations. Documented experiences are different from person to person, and from session to session. One comment that I hear across the board from all my clients is that they are always very hungry or thirsty post–healing sesh!

WHO BENEFITS FROM CRYSTAL HEALING?

Anyone can benefit, as long as they come into a session with a positive attitude and an open heart and mind. No agenda, no expectations, no cynicism. These can be the biggest barriers to crystal healing having a lasting effect. There isn't a one-size-fits-all recipe, and the treatment is always a bespoke experience.

What gets affected or recalibrated in the physical, mental, emotional, and spiritual body during a crystal healing session?

1. *Emotional:* Stabilize moods, enhance self-esteem
2. *Mental:* Enhanced clarity and creativity; increased focus and awareness; lessening of unhealthy behaviors; relief from addictions and thought patterns like negative self-talk and limiting beliefs

3. *Physical:* Relief from stress, sleep problems, panic attacks, chronic fatigue, anxiety, infertility, migraines, joint pain, digestive disorders, chronic or severe illnesses

4. *Spiritual:* Feeling centered, peaceful, and harmonious; greater acceptance of others

FINDING YOUR "POWER STONES"

Our ancestors had to gather stones and crystals from riverbanks, beaches, forests, caves, and mountain trails. We can still do this today, but we also have a more convenient option: journeying to our friendly neighborhood metaphysical store to pick out the right crystal for what ails us. Choosing the right crystals—your "Power Stones," the ones that you feel the greatest connection with—is actually really easy and intuitive. You don't have to be a shaman or a Reiki master to do it. A stone is

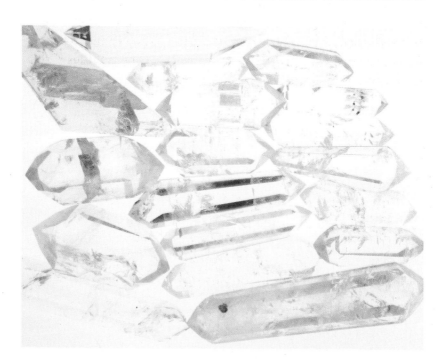

the right stone if it speaks to you. If you walk into a metaphysical store and find yourself drawn to a particular stone, if that stone is screaming, *"Pick me, pick me,"* then you should be open to considering it one of your Power Stones. Your Power Stones might also come to you through healing practitioners and friends, or you might find one on a hike or after an extensive Google search. Power Stones can be used in a multitude of ways, and the reason you are initially drawn to a particular stone may change over time.

Different crystal types carry different vibrations and have different uses, which is why they each have an individualized purpose when we work with them. However, there are certain stones, referred to as *master healing stones,* that are must-haves. And these are the ideal stones to start your crystal collection with if you are a beginner. Clear Quartz is *the* primary Master Healer. It's a multipurpose healing stone, and it has the ability to amplify the energy of just about any situation. Because of its versatility, it is the single most beneficial stone you can introduce into your life. Clear Quartz is like the neutral that goes with any outfit—I call it the "black skinny jean" of the crystal kingdom! The other master healing stones mentioned have a diverse range of properties and uses. These stones cover all the basics:

The Master Healing Stones

Amethyst

Black Obsidian

Carnelian

Citrine

Clear Quartz

Rose Quartz

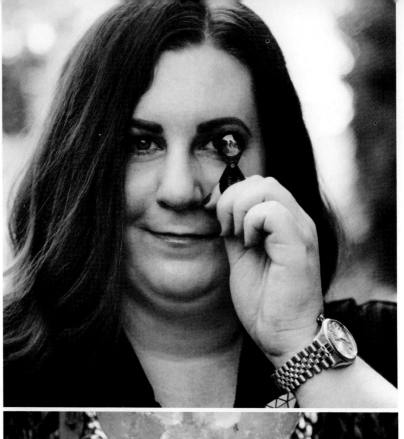
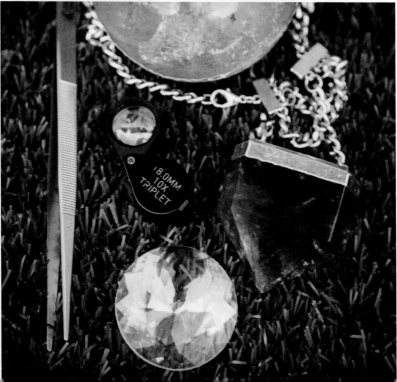

A Lesson in Crystal Basics with Joy the Gemologist

I'D LIKE TO INTRODUCE STYLE RITUALS' HOUSE GEMOLOGIST, Joyanne "Joy" Prebyl, a gem expert and graduate of the Gemological Institute of America. Read on for the nitty-gritty facts from Joy on the most commonly asked crystal questions.

How do crystals form?

Crystals are formed from chemical elements inside the earth's crust, usually over the course of thousands, millions, or billions of years. Crystals all form in the same way: atoms come together to form a uniform cluster with a distinctive way of locking new atoms into a three-dimensional pattern called a crystal structure, which repeats again and again. A crystal's unique characteristics (shape, size, color, clarity) are determined by its atomic structure.

Where do crystals form?

Every country on Earth has a selection of minerals under the ground, although some places are hotbeds for various types of stones. Crystals need very specific conditions, and space, to grow. A crystal starts out microscopically small and expands from there. Crystals can grow in tightly packed earth, spacious rock caves, or pools of mineral rich water. Crystals can also grow on rock walls, on other crystals, and on dust particles. The length of time it takes crystals to form varies depending on the chemical composition and temperature changes.

What's the difference between a rock and a stone?

Nothing, really! This is a "you say to-may-to, I say to-mah-to" sort of situation. Rocks and stones are composed of minerals (natural, inorganic substances with a chemical composition). Rocks and stones are both aggregates (a group of tightly packed crystals). Lapis lazuli, for example, is a beautiful "rock" that is commonly turned into jewelry. It is an aggregate of several minerals, including but not limited to calcite, lazurite, and pyrite.

What is the difference between a crystal and a gemstone?

To be considered a gemstone, a mineral must be considered rare, beautiful, and long-lasting. Most minerals form as crystals (solid matter with atoms arranged in a regular, repeating, three-dimensional pattern called a crystal structure). One fun fact an educator taught me is that crystal composition is the only difference between graphite (what's used in pencils) and a diamond. Many crystals, like Rose Quartz, are beautiful, but not necessarily valuable.

What's the deal with igneous, metamorphous, and sedimentary rocks?

All natural gemstones can be found in one of these three basic categories (which you may vaguely remember learning about in high school science class). *Igneous* rocks (ex., tourmaline, aquamarine, moonstone) are produced by the cooling of magma, or molten rock, from volcanoes. *Sedimentary* rocks (ex., turquoise, opal, malachite) are typically formed when water erosion breaks down minerals and redeposits them into compact layers, which grow with the earth as it shifts and moves to create new rock. *Metamorphic* rocks (ex., emerald, ruby, sapphire) form when pressure and heat causes preexisting igneous, sedimentary, or metamorphic rocks to change and become cemented together during the earth's shifting.

Can you explain the differences between natural and man-made gemstones?

Natural gemstones are those created by our magnificent Mother Earth without any human help. *Man-made* gemstones fall under two categories: synthetic and imitation. *Synthetic* stones are created in a lab to have primarily the same properties, crystal structure, and crystal composition as natural stones. So these gems are totally real, but they are not naturally grown from Mother Earth. Lab-grown diamonds are an example of synthetic gemstones. *Imitation* stones are made from a variety of materials to look almost identical to a natural gem, but they do not have the same chemical composition. Fun fact: Rubies are the most synthesized gem on the market, so be careful when purchasing!

What are organic and inorganic gems?

Organic gems are those formed by or of living things (plants or animals). Examples of organic gems are amber, coral, pearl, and ivory. Inorganic gems, those made up of minerals, are everything else: topaz, emerald, diamond, ruby, etc.

MY SIGNATURE SAUCE: THE STYLE RITUALS INTUITIVE CRYSTAL READING METHOD

My crystal practice is a bit of a pupu platter of spiritual modalities, based on what I have learned from my spiritual teachers, my own experiences, and by observing what resonates most with my clients, who I always say are my greatest teachers. In my past life in fashion, I was doing something quite different from my present-day occupation, but in an oddly similar way. As a stylist, I would present visual information to my clients around coming trends, with the idea of anticipating what was coming in the next season, or in the future. I would build a fashion-friendly vision board filled with magazine tearsheets and strewn with trinkets from my overseas trending-travel trips in order to bring a style story to life. Now, instead of building trend boards for fashion and beauty brands, I combine my style sense with my spiritual intuition to construct visual narratives of a client's past, present, and future using tarot cards and crystals.

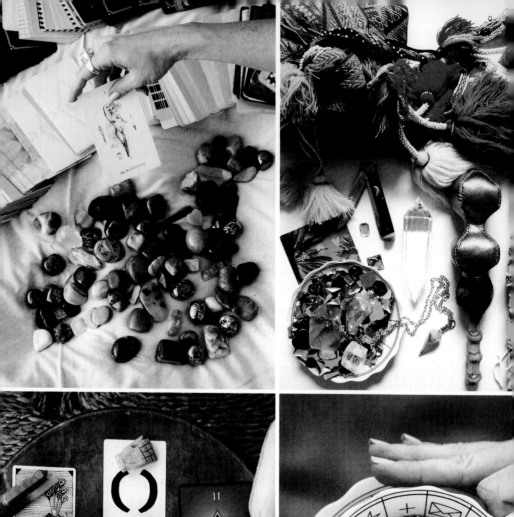
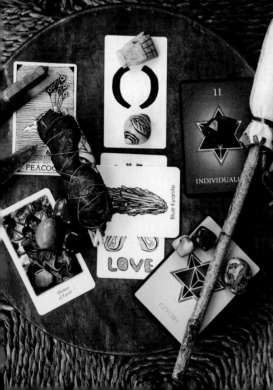
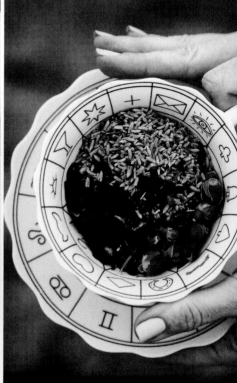

I'm a "go big or go home" type of girl, so I never use just one tarot deck or one crystal in a reading. On any given day, I'll have dozens of different decks and crystals mixed into a spread that I individually create for a client, and none of it's random. I choose each crystal deliberately to speak to the potential subjects we'll be discussing. My reading style is untraditional, but it's very effective—according to my clients!

Within my tarot stack, you'll find cards that represent goddesses and oracles, mantras and positive affirmations, numerology and astrology, past lives and spirit animals, along with cards from traditional Rider-Waite tarot decks. The crystals I choose for a reading cover all the typical subjects that you might discuss over cocktails with a close friend: love, money, family, emotions, manifestation, life changes, fashion choices, moving, and job security. Once my tarot cards have been laid out in a spread, I then blow on the crystals with my breath and ask my clients to blow with their breath on the chosen crystals in my hands. I shake them a bit and then toss them over the top of the cards like throwing dice in Vegas. This is my modern-day version of geomancy, or "stone throwing." I like to keep my bag of tricks interesting, and to have a dynamic palette of images and objects in front of me. No two readings are ever alike! The framework of my reading style is unusual, out-of-the-box, and definitely unorthodox, but I've found my divination methods to be very effective. And I always send my clients home with some Mystical Homework and a crystal gift bag (obviously!).

WHAT'S IN MY MEDICINE BAG?

A medicine bag is not always a "bag" in the traditional sense. Native American shamans use a purse or necklace-like bag, while South American shamans and shamans from other lineages around the world use a container that is relevant to or reflective of their cultural traditions. Regardless of the type of vessel or design, a medicine bag is filled with healing items, spiritual tools, and sacred talismans, and the practice of carrying one has been embraced by shamans around the world for centuries. The contents of a medicine bag will vary from one shaman to the next, but within the Peruvian shamanic tradition, a full medicine bag, or *mesa* (which means "table" or "high plateau" in Spanish), contains thirteen stones known as *khuyas*. A shaman uses the contents of his or her bag to perform hands-on healings and ceremonial rites, and to teach and provide council to others. A shaman may lay the *khuya* over the afflicted chakras on a client's body to allow an energetic healing to take place, with the participation of the client, the shaman, and the Spirit Guides. This is a team effort, so the client must be open and willing to participate in the healing to see change happen.

Many of the *khuyas* in my medicine bag come from energetic hotspots that I've visited around the world. And each of my thirteen stones has a unique story behind it. I also carry other small talismans that inspire me.

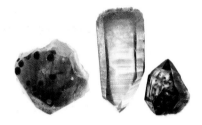

CHOOSING YOUR CRYSTALS

"You don't choose the crystal. The crystal chooses you!"

Crystals all have different capabilities and powers. Certain stones are ideal for healing the body, some are best for tapping into your intuition, others are suited for working on emotional issues. The crystal you need will speak to you! When you first come into contact with your crystal, you may experience any of the following sensations: the stone may get hot in your hand, you may feel tingles into your arm, or you may feel a third-eye buzz. You may also "just know," or feel, that a crystal you encounter is a good fit. Trust your intuition. If a crystal doesn't feel quite right in your hand, then go with your gut—it's not meant for you.

GETTING STARTED

Before you begin to amass your crystal collection, do a personal inventory of what's up for you, and ask yourself these simple questions:

- What mental, emotional, spiritual, or physical issues would you like to address right now? Once you've pinpointed these topics, refer to "A Lesson in Color Psychology" (page 52) and "The Top 20 Stones Every Girl Needs in Her Arsenal" (page 59) for advice on the right crystal types and colors for what ails you.

- What's your budget? Be aware of how much you want to spend on your crystals, and shop with intention. Pick what you can afford and start out small before buying bigger or more expensive pieces.

MEET 'N' GREET: ADVICE ON PERUSING YOUR LOCAL METAPHYSICAL SHOP

In my travels, I meet crystal vendors from all over the world, and I source my stones from crystal experts I trust. It's not practical for everyone to journey to a gem mine and hand-pick their own stones, but your local metaphysical shop is the next best thing. Take the time to meet and talk to the store owners, and ask them about where they source their stones and if they can fill you in on the history of a stone you are interested in. This is what I do. You want ethically sourced stones, and those with the most positive, clean, clear energies possible. Knowing the lineage of a crystal is a lot like knowing where your meat or your eggs come from. Free-range and farm-to-table, right?

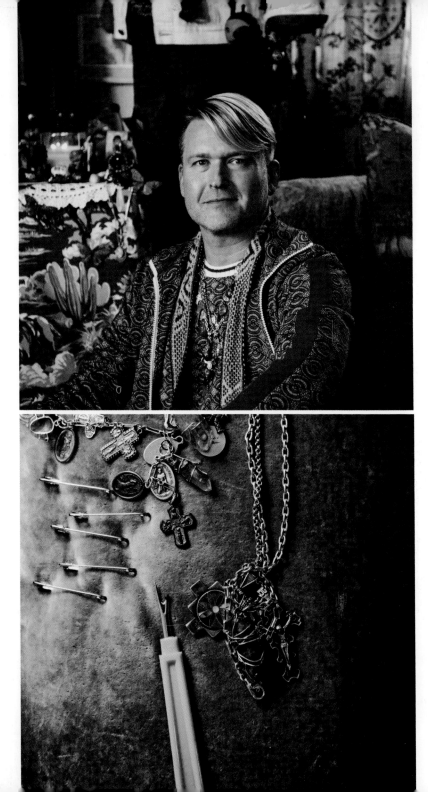

Interview with John Murphy

LET'S MEET ANOTHER FASHION STYLIST TURNED SHAMAN, John Murphy, and see how he incorporates crystals into his career. Although we didn't get into his personal closet, we did visit where he keeps all the sparkle: his Nashville-based agency, Corazon Creative.

Who have you styled?

My clients have included Britney Spears, Garth Brooks, Kenny Chesney, Brad Paisley, Rascal Flatts, Runaway June, Chase Bryant, Dustin Lynch, Parmalee, Easton Corbin, John Hardy, and Jason Aldean and his wife, Brittany.

How did you get into the fashion biz?

My first fashion assistant job was in Nashville in 1997 on a Garth Brooks video. I assisted for a year and then moved to LA. My business grew bigger after I moved to LA because I became a West Coast fashion representative for the country music community. I ended up moving back to Nashville to build a closer relationship with my clients. I have anywhere from twenty-five to thirty clients at a time. I toured with Rascal Flatts for five years, and you can always find me backstage at the Academy of Country Music awards and the CMT awards or the Grammys. With my clients, I would work with a creative team to build album packages and shoot music videos, photoshoots, commercials, and ad campaigns.

How did you get into crystals?

As a child, I would find rocks in nature. I had girl cousins who had crystal necklaces, but growing up in a small Midwestern town, it wasn't masculine to have crystals, so I hid them under my bed. I would also sketch perfume bottles (which looked like crystals) as a kid. I decorated my whole room in high school in Santa Fe style (which felt very shamanic). As I got into my country music career, which at the time was still a very "straight" and traditionally masculine industry, I embodied my love of crystals by living vicariously through my clients on the red carpet. I got to add rhinestones to an ensemble or fancy pocket squares. Until I started studying shamanism, I had no idea how shamanic what I was doing was—the rhinestones and sacred-geometry patterns that are laid in on country music shirts, the embroidery of shamanic archetypes.

When did you go "full crystal"?

Three years ago, I started seeing my first energy healer in Nashville. After several sessions with her, I met you, started reading books on shamanism, and started hanging out at Cosmic Connections (Nashville's go-to crystal store). I also went on a soul-searching vacation, which gave me the space and clarity to "see" myself again. I was ready to become the full expression of myself, not just a shell or version of myself. I also started my crystal collection. I have a neatly labeled collection of stones and am learning all the meanings as well as what I am vibing off with my experiences and those of my clients.

What's Corazon Creative?

It's a full-service referral agency. It's a one-stop shop for industry people who aren't familiar with the Nashville market and need to tap into the resources. Instead of flying teams in from New York or LA, we can find talent here for their projects. I've been a stylist for twenty years, and I was ready to become more of a mentor and guide to the younger generation of people working in the entertainment industry. It was time for my career to evolve, so I blended my shamanic training with my stylist skills, and now my clients come over and get a suit fitting and a chakra cleanse, or a dress fitting with a curated set of crystals. Besides traditional agency services, we also offer mindfulness resources for our clients. We build a safe place where they can voice their interests or needs, whether it be about a campaign or a crystal. An industry Jiffy-Lube for your inside and outside!

How do you fuse together styling and shamanism?

I didn't know it early on in my career, but I was working with all these shamanic elements! I am now conscious of how shaman-y the decoration within country music is; stones like hematite and turquoise to decorate shirts, and southwestern motifs and floral prints that echo sacred symbolisms. When doing a clothing pull for a client's event or shoot, I choose way less clothing, because I use my intuition and divination skills to pick three great dresses I know are all front-runners instead of fifty for a fitting.

How do religion and shamanism work together for you?

My faith in the Catholic church had been diminished due to their beliefs around homosexuality. As much as I love the foundational principles of Catholicism, I didn't want to go to church and be told I was going to go to hell for who I loved. Exploring shamanism and other belief systems restored my faith in the founding principles of Christianity as opposed to diminishing them. A common misconception is that shamanism is correlated with witchcraft. It's all about honoring oneself, nature, and everyone around you—basically, it's echoing the first two commandments, "Do unto others as you would like done to you" and "Love you neighbor as yourself." I'm not trying to get all political, *but* unfortunately, the origins of what Christianity was meant to be got manipulated by people in power. If Christianity returned to its purest form, I believe it would have a resurgence. In its current state, we see a decline. If people acknowledged change and acknowledged that things are going on outside of the little boxes they live in, we would all be better off. Acknowledge it, even if you don't understand it—"I see you, I may not like it, but I see you." We can really start to look at each other with love in our hearts instead of looking at people as being black, white, gay, straight, etc.

If you were a crystal, which crystal would you be?

Aqua Aura Quartz, because of the color. Its everything I want to be: bright, sparkly, rainbow, iridescent, and misshapen, but perfect.

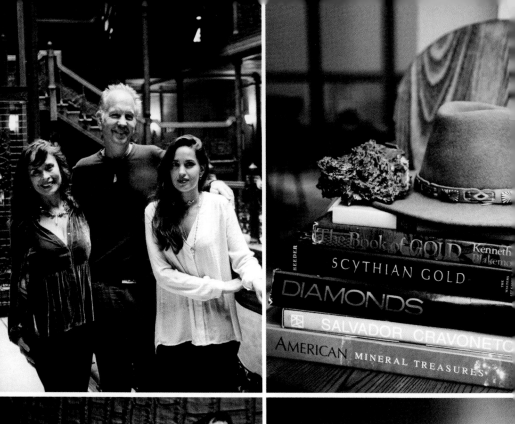

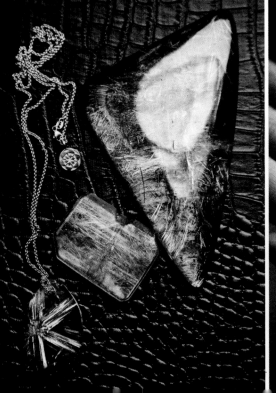

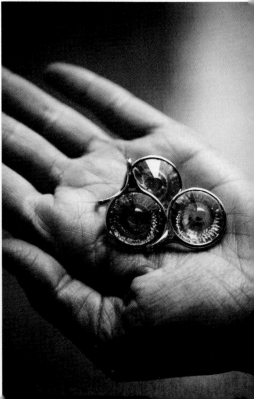

Respect Your Crystals: Interview with Brian, Kendra, and Quendi Cook

BRIAN IS A GEOLOGIST BY TRADE and has been in the gem business his entire adult life. He consults with major names in the fashion and gem industry, including Harry Winston, Cartier, Tiffany, and Swarovski. He consults on all things with his company, including ethical gem sourcing, selling stones to designers and design houses, cutting gems, and even mining them. Brian works all over the world but mostly in Brazil. He is known for his work with exotic and rare gemstones and is one of the pioneers in his industry striving to build a sustainable business model.

What is your opinion on taking the stones out of the ground?

Some people think taking minerals out of the earth is doing something wrong to the earth. My first response is, they aren't going anywhere. They're just interacting on another energy level, with humans. More crystals are being formed as we speak, and through tectonic processes they will eventually get pushed to the surface. Technically speaking, heat, pressure, and temperature move volatiles through the earth, which form the veins, so to say, of the earth. The earth's crust is constantly going through

a distillation process from the buildup of heat and pressure. Eventually "the veins" migrate off in different directions into pockets and bubbles, and crystals form. When removing the crystals from the ground, we look at it like a distilling process. Our company motto at Nature's Geometry is "We are bringing the light to the surface," in an ethical way.

What happens when you find a crystal (especially large or rare ones)?

Everyone, from miner to dealer, partners on and benefits from the process; everyone receives a cut of the profits and recognition.

Does mining crystals energetically disrupt the harmonious nature of the earth?

We are not removing them from our global matrix; we are just moving them. It's a natural evolutionary process to work with stones. They are tools for spiritual development. Changing which layer of the earth they are on is a natural evolutionary process. If you look at the animal kingdom, which we are a part of, we are made up of minerals just like crystals are. We are just giant crystals. It's a bigger question of running out of *all* resources—metal, wood, etc.

What about ethical and responsible gem sourcing?

It's a big subject in our industry. The jewelry business is coming to this late in the game compared to the coffee, food, chocolate, and textile industries. I speak all around the world on this subject. Our industry needs to deal with this, but it's complicated, because it is global, made of all kinds of different cultural mores, and one of the oldest industries in the world. It is also based on cloak-and-dagger policies and secrecy, which is the opposite of transparency. Traceability and transparency of gem sources are needed and wanted, as people want to know what they are putting their money into. Stones actually help support people all over the world. If we can improve what people are receiving when they buy stones, we can change the game. We especially want to empower women by teaching them lapidary skills.

What made you get into the ethical side of the stone industry?

It's my personal passion.

Why are people so drawn to gems?

Crystals have always been a source of magic and power with shamans and energy workers, as well as symbols of wealth, and they're known to have healing properties. Power and magic exist within these crystals. The more power you have, the more precious gems you are going to have!

What gems do you specialize in?

Paraíba tourmaline, golden rutilated quartz (also known in the Chinese tradition as "golden needle"), spessartine garnet, pegmatite, and emeralds. I am known as "the Rutile King." I supplemented my income in college by importing stones from South America. I also mine epitaxial crystals, which are the same crystals that are used in technology. (Epitaxial means the crystals of one substance grow on the crystal face of another substance.)

Gem Legacy

The family that gems together, ha-ha . . . I have uncles and great-uncles who came out west as gold prospectors. My brother is one of the top geologists in the world. I diverted from regular geology and into the magical realms of crystals and gems because I am an artist. I am an expert in gemstones. Kendra, my wife, is a Brazilian intuitive-healer who has published several books on gems. Quendi, my daughter, is the bridge between people in our business. She helps run our family business on all levels, from mining logistics to our lines of jewelry, Wheel of Light and Aromajewels.

Are there ethical standards in gems as in the clothing industry?

Environmental pollution, child labor, fair pay, and safe working conditions are being accounted for already. One of the biggest barriers is transparency, because there is such a long chain of custody with a gem. You could find a gem in Brazil that will get sent to China for cutting and processing and then be sold a few times through trade shows and private buyers, before finally moving on to a designer or design house and then to the consumer. (On average, a gem will be sold two or three times before it even gets to a designer.) The levels of standard and conditions are variable. The biggest cutting centers are in China, India, and Bangkok. The majority of people buying stones from the mine are Chinese.

What are the challenges and issues with ethical gem-sourcing initiatives?

Funding is the number one issue, but we are very close to the time of things turning over because the industry needs to change. Michael Kowalski, the former head of Tiffany, is looking to spearhead this initiative. We spend billions of dollars on advertising, so why not promote this, too? It's a story the whole industry can share.

What do people want to know about their gemstones?

"Is there child labor, where do things come from, what are the conditions, what am I paying for?" Awareness around stones blew up with Leonardo DiCaprio's *Blood Diamond* movie. Gems are sprinkled all over the planet, and they are mostly found in remote areas and mined by poor people in those areas. That is considered "artisanal" mining. Like their meat, eggs, or clothing, people now want to know where their gems are coming from and that they are ethically harvested under fair labor practices. I am a member of the Geneva Coalition and sit alongside other members like Chanel, Louis Vuitton, and Cartier to discuss, educate, and initiate how we get the aforementioned ideas into practice.

Tell us about your amazing initiative in Brazil.

Most big companies are working from the top down with CSR initiatives. I am working from the bottom up with my project in Bahia, Brazil. We are bringing value through product by opening a lapidary school to create skilled laborers and biodynamic organic farming for the community so that food is sustainable. By investing in sustainable activity, we are creating a responsible ecosystem and traceability. In 1983, I was the first foreigner they had ever seen. We lived within the community and in 1987 the village elder and shaman said to me, "Are you ready to buy the pyramid?" The land remained as a preserve for many years. The mine didn't become legal until a year and a half ago. It took thirteen years to get the permits. There are three thousand miners who have been working the land for hundreds of years. We now have electricity, and everyone has a cell phone. When we first went, there was no electricity. The mine is under a giant pyramid covered in greenery that had been struck by lightning at one point and the tip was blown off. We are located in the remote town of Remédios, which means "medicine." My legacy would be to get this initiative set up and to use this as an example of a sustainable investment model around the world for abandoned and new mines.

Did you know Marcel Vogel (former IBM research scientist and founder of Psychic Research Inc.)?

Yes. Kendra started making models of the Seven Crystal Systems in the

1980s and came up with a collection called "Star Gems." Kendra knew she needed to go to a scientist to help her with what she was creating. When we moved back to the states in 1989, we got in touch with Marcel. We went to his lab and shared our idea. Marcel said, "Oh, you've got something here, but you must put the design in line with your own axis . . . your own spinal column."

He helped us create pendants taking into account what he had told us.

If you were a crystal, which crystal will you be?

BRIAN: Paraíba Tourmaline
KENDRA: Quartz Crystal, because it is full spectrum, reflects the light, and is versatile
QUENDI: Emerald

FINDING YOUR CRYSTALS

I SEE YOU!

As you are perusing the shelves, let your eyes do the work. You may stumble upon a crystal that you just can't pass up. You may keep coming back to one particular stone, holding it, and rereading what Google has to say about its powers. It may not be the biggest, prettiest, or most sparkly, or the stone you thought you came in to buy. But none of that matters—that crystal is meant for you! This is a moment of trust.

I FEEL YOU!

Close your eyes and take one big clearing breath. Let your hand hover about one inch over each potential crystal you are looking to purchase. Your hand may get hot, or you may feel tingles in your arm. This is a YES! Compare it to the chemistry you may have felt on a good first date . . . there were fireworks! Another approach is running your hand through a pile, basket, or tray of crystals. One will inevitably find its way into your hand, and you won't be able to let go. In order to confirm that a crystal is a yes, you may get that body tingle or sensation. The way I perform this practice is by always putting the crystal in my *left* hand, because when we talk about the flow of energy channels, this is the feminine or receiving side of the body. Then I wait for the tingle!

Finger Dowsing

Finger dowsing is another technique used for choosing crystals, based on the idea that your body has a particular energy field that reacts with external fields of energy. Through finger dowsing, your intuition is going to communicate with your fingers:

1. Loop your thumb and pointer finger together as shown.

2. Slip your other thumb and pointer finger together through the loop and close them tightly, like you are making two "OK" hand signals. Hold your hands over the crystal in question and ask yourself, *Is this crystal for me?*

3. If your loop holds, the answer is yes. If you feel it pulling apart, the answer is no.

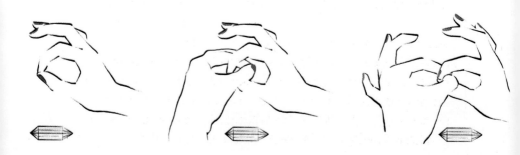

Invoke the Power of a Pendulum

You can also use a pendulum to find your crystal. Pendulums can be made of crystal, wood, or metal, and they typically hang from a metal chain or a string. The most common combination is a single-terminated crystal point on a six- to eight-inch metal chain (like the drawing shown here). If you are a beginner, I recommend buying a pendulum in person at a metaphysical shop, asking the shop owner for help, and taking your pendulum for a test drive before you buy it.

Once you have your pendulum, here are instructions for using it to choose a crystal:

1. Begin by taking a few deep breaths to ground yourself. Sit comfortably somewhere and make sure your arms and legs are uncrossed. You can rest your elbow on a table in front of you, allowing the pendulum to swing freely, or you can hold your arm in a horizontal position, again allowing your pendulum to swing freely. Continue to breathe with intention to keep your energy channel open.

2. Establish "yes" and "no" with your pendulum: Hold the pendulum loosely in your nondominant hand between your fingers and thumb. Allow the pendulum to hang and ask a yes-or-no question, like, "Is my name _____?" and give your real name. Pay attention to the way the pendulum swings—this is your "yes" answer. The pendulum may swing clockwise, counterclockwise, or elliptically, or it may even shake slightly and pull down toward the ground. You must interpret as best you can. Next, ask, "Is my name _____?" and give an incorrect answer. Watch how the pendulum swings, and this direction is your "no" answer.

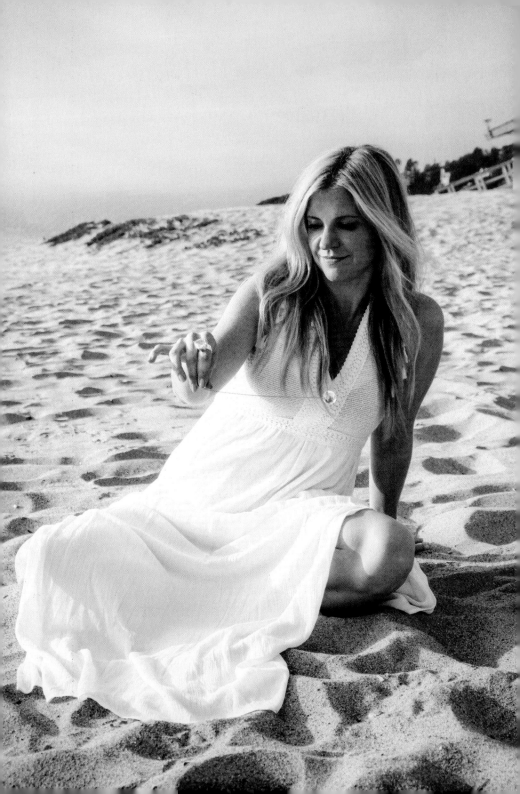

3. Now that you've established "yes" and "no," hold your pendulum over the crystal in question and ask, "Is this the crystal for me?" Watch the way the pendulum moves, and you have your answer!

Become a Human Pendulum!

Forgot your pendulum at home? No problem. You can use your body to find your magic rock by using the kinesthetic "Sway Test":

1. Stand up and relax your shoulders and your knees. Take a few deep yoga breaths.
2. Figure out which way your body sways when an answer is "yes" versus "no" by asking yourself the name question again. When you ask, "Is my name _____?" saying your real name, you should feel your body sway slightly forward or backward. This is your "yes" direction. Now repeat the question with an incorrect name. Your body will again sway forward or backward—this is your "no."
3. Practice until you notice a definite sway. Now you can use this technique to pick crystals, as well as beauty products, fruits at the grocery store—you name it! This will give you excellent insight into what your body wants or wants to avoid in any situation. (P.S. Don't forget to hold the product in your nondominant hand while asking!)

CHAKRA CLEANSE: THE GREEN JUICE OF ENERGY HEALING

One of my favorite forms of crystal healing is the Chakra Cleanse, which aligns, revitalizes, and focuses the body for an overall system boost. Please note: Chakra cleansing is a very powerful method of cleansing unwanted energy from the physical and energetic body. I am going to give you the 101 on how I work in a session, followed by a starter version to try on your own at home. However, if you would like to learn how to do this for others in a professional setting, I ask that you train with an accredited healer or organization that will provide you with the right setting, tools, and education to truly understand the breadth and depth of this practice.

But first, you need to understand what a chakra is, where your various chakras are, and what color coordinates with the energy each one carries.

CHAKRAS 101

WHAT IS A CHAKRA?

Over three thousand years ago, people living in present-day Tibet and India discovered energy portal points on the body. This interconnected web of energy points has become known as the chakra system. On a macro level, our chakras are personal portals into the vast and inter-connected energy system of the universe. On a micro level, they are a link between our physical and subtle energy bodies. Each chakra corresponds to a specific point on the body, and they act as gateways or energy exchange points, allowing energy in and out like a river dam. Chakras are often described as circular, wheel-like, tornado-shaped, or glowing balls of energy. And they spin! Healthy chakras spin clockwise, while unhealthy chakras spin counterclockwise, or can become broken-down or misshapen. Chakras can become blocked by negative thought patterns, emotional issues, physical toxins, etc.

Different spiritual traditions work with different versions of the chakra system, and therefore different healers work with different numbers of chakras. Many ancient Eastern healing modalities and spiritual tradi-tions believe we have as many as 114 chakras, and an additional 72,000 *nadis*, or energy channels, where vital energy, or prana, moves! The twelve-chakra system (seven main chakras in the body and five outside the body in the energetic field) is most commonly embraced by contemporary healers and energy workers. I know, it's a bit confusing, but don't stress. To keep things simple, in this book we are only going to focus on the first seven chakras. Phew!

THE SEVEN-CHAKRA SYSTEM

Each chakra point "vibrates" to a different color frequency and has a specific connection to the way that we function on a physical, mental, emotional, and spiritual level. Crystals that "match" a chakra color carry healing properties for that particular chakra, and I place crystals on the corresponding chakra in my healing sessions.

1st Chakra—Root Chakra

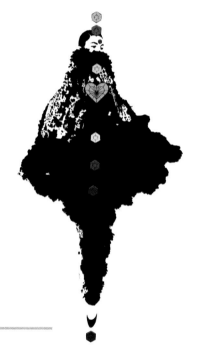

Color: Red
Location: The base of the spine, genitals
Crystal Pairing: Fire Agate, Fire Opal, Garnet, Red Brecciated Jasper, Red Tiger's Eye, Ruby
The Heals: anger, blood ailments, bravery, energy, exhilaration, grounding, health safety, improving circulation, love, money, power, primalness, primal self, protection, reproduction and fertility, sex organs, sexuality, strength, survival needs

2nd Chakra—Sacral Chakra

Color: Orange/Peach
Location: Just below the belly button

Crystal Pairing: Amber, Carnelian, Mookaite, Orange Optical Calcite, Peach Aura Quartz, Sunstone
The Heals: action, community, creativity, digestion, emotions, feelings, freshness, immune system, menopause, menstruation, ovaries, self-motivation, vitality, weight

3rd Chakra—Solar Plexus Chakra

Color: Yellow
Location: Where the rib cage meets, above the belly button and below the chest
Crystal Pairing: Iron Pyrite, Citrine, Honey Calcite, Yellow Topaz, Yellow Jasper
The Heals: attracting money, authority, awareness of tasks, caution, courage, digestion, eating disorders, energy, harmony, happiness, increased alertness, intellect, liver, lymphatic system, mental clarity, metabolism, new projects, optimism, personal identity, personal power, relationships, self-confidence, self-esteem, solidify vigor, stomach, vision, zest

4th Chakra—Heart Chakra

Color: Green or Pink
Location: The center of the chest
Green Crystal Pairing: Aventurine, Amazonite, Emerald, Fluorite, Green Calcite, Hiddenite, Jade, Malachite, Moldavite, Moss Agate, Ocean Jasper
Pink Crystal Pairing: Chrysoprase, Kunzite, Morganite, Pink Botswana Agate, Pink Manganocalcite, Pink Chalcedony, Pink Tourmaline, Rose Quartz, Unakite
The Heals: addictions, compassion, female hormones and reproductive issues, friendship, heart, heart conditions, kindness, love, lungs,

panic attacks, psychological issues, respiratory issues, self-love, sleep disorders, stress-induced illness, worthiness

5th Chakra—Throat Chakra

Color: Light Blue
Location: The center of the throat/clavicle bone
Crystal Pairing: Angelite, Aqua Aura Quartz, Blue Apatite, Blue Kyanite, Blue Lace Agate, Blue Onyx, Blue Tourmaline, Celestite, Chalcopyrite, Chrysocolla, Lapis Lazuli, Larimar, Sodalite, Turquoise,
The Heals: ancestors, angels, blood pressure, calming, communication, creative expression fluidity, headache and eye problems, honesty, intuition, invisible helpers like Spirit Guides, issues, lower mouth/teeth/gums, meditation, peaceful, purity, soothing, stress relief, throat, thyroid, truth, transformation

6th Chakra—Third Eye Chakra

Color: Indigo
Location: The middle of the forehead between your eyes
Crystal Pairing: Amethyst, Blue Goldstone, Blue Tiger's Eye, Blue Tourmaline, Fluorite, Iolite, Lapis Lazuli
The Heals: amplification of senses, devotion, evolutionary gain, foresight, future-seeing, higher schools of thought, honor, inner-knowing, insightful, insight, intuition jaw, mouth, perception, potential, psychic gifts, spiritual wisdom, telepathy, tongue

7th Chakra—Crown Chakra

Color: Violet or Gold
Location: The top of the head

Crystal Pairing: Amethyst, Ametrine, Charoite, Fluorite, Iron Pyrite, Jade, Lepidolite, Smoky Elestial Quartz, Sugilite, Super Seven

The Heals: addiction, astral projection, bridging between two places, connection to "God," consciousness, headaches, hyperactivity, keeping away physical toxicity (people or environments), leadership, nervous disorders, phobias and psychological disorders, royalty, sinuses, wisdom

WHAT ABOUT OTHER CRYSTAL COLORS AND THE CHAKRAS?

Black, brown, and ***gray/silver*** crystals all work with the Root Chakra and the 10th chakra, or Earth Star Chakra, which is below the feet.

Black Crystal Pairing: Apache Tears, Black Agate, Black Jade, Black Kyanite, Black Moonstone, Black Obsidian, Black Tourmaline, Chinese Writing Rock, Hypersthene, Jet, Onyx, Shungite, Snowflake Obsidian, Tektite

The Heals: being introverted, control, cyclic endings, fears of physical harm, going inwards, grief and depression, grounding, invisibility, knowledge, masculinity, pain relief, panic attacks, protection, protector when doing spiritual work, self-doubt, shield from EMFs, shields from mental/physical/emotional and energetic traumas, silence, stillness, well-being, X-rays and chemotherapy, yang energy

Brown Crystal Pairing: Aragonite, Banded Agate, Boulder Opal, Brown Stripe Jasper, Desert Rose, Fossils, Lionskin, Montana Agate, Petrified Wood, Smoky Quartz, Stromatolite, Tiger's Eye

The Heals: authenticity, bowels and large intestines, dedication, easing stress, honesty, one day at a time, sensible, slow and steady, stability, strength for the emotional body, strong yet subtle, vitality

Gray/Silver Crystal Pairing: Botswana Agate, Gibeon Meteorite, Hematite, Platinum Quartz

The Heals: compliant, conservative, cools intensity, detachment, efficiency, escape, isolation, lone wolves, maturity, mental illness, narrow-mindedness, neutrality, non-invasive, practicality, retreat, security, temper avoidance

White/clear crystals work with the 8th, 9th, 11th, and 12th chakras, which reside over the top of the head.

White crystal pairing: Angel Aura Quartz, Clear Quartz, Dream Quartz, Girasol, Herkimer Diamond, Howlite, Milky Quartz, Moonstone, Opal, Opalite, Scolecite, Selenite, Snow Quartz

The Heals: a "bridge" between points A and B, amplification, balance, breast and womb problems, cleanliness, expectant mothers, general health, goddess energy, innocence, mental clarity, purification, radiance, spiritual connection, unity, yin energy

THE STYLE RITUALS SIGNATURE CHAKRA CLEANSE

1. As I begin a Chakra Cleanse, the very first thing I do is to open a "sacred space," creating a safe and strong energetic "container" for my client's healing. I open what shamans call "The Four Directions," and I also call all my helping Spirit Guides into the room, as well as my client's Spirit Guides. Once I feel the space is ready, we can get started. Every healer does this space-opening process differently, but it is one of the most important steps in the process.

2. Next I like to start a dialogue with my client about their lifestyle and their needs, to get a full picture of where they are currently.

I ask questions like: What are you trying to achieve from our work together today? What does an average day look like for you? What do you do for a living? How have your health, diet, sleep, and exercise patterns been? Do you have any preexisting conditions? What other healing modalities are you working with? Do you have any opposition to sage smoke or allergies to topical oils? Are there any crystal energies you are overly sensitive to? When was the last time you had an energy healing? And the *most* important question: Do I have permission to work with you today?

3. Then I choose my crystals and stones. Different crystal colors, shapes, and textures have special meanings, and these can play into my decision about what to work with. I use my right brain and *flex my intuitive muscle* by going with the crystals I feel most drawn to. Next I check in with my left brain and do a cross-check of the crystals I've picked against my training in crystals according to what each stone traditionally represents. If you do this yourself, you will find that, in most cases, you will have intuitively picked a crystal that works for what ails you without even meaning to. The main stones that I work with in a Chakra Cleanse come from my medicine bag, and I add other crystals as I see fit.

4. My client lies on their back on a flat surface: a yoga mat, blanket, massage table, bed, etc. I ask if they need a pillow for under the head, knees, or back, and if they need any extra floor padding. The space should be quiet, comfortable, and temperate.

5. The stones may be used alone or accompanied by other healing instruments. I am a big fan of accessories, so I always have my entire shamanic arsenal at my side: sacred herbs, oils, rattles, drums, feathers, and a crystal bowl. I work completely intuitively, so I won't know until I am in the moment what accompanying healing "ally" I will need during the session. I am also a Reiki master, so I like to infuse hands-on healing into my sessions as well.

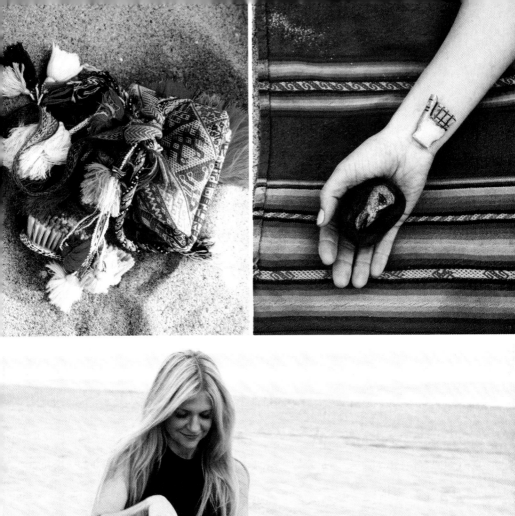
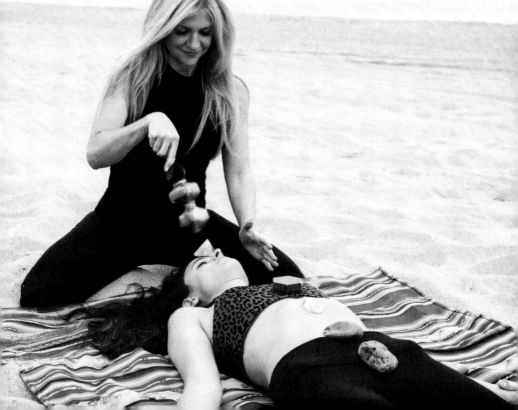

6. I place the crystals on my client's body, working either from feet to head or from head to feet, depending on which way I want the energy to move. If I want energy to move from "sky to earth" (head to feet), I'll arrange my crystal points toward the client's "south," or Root Chakra. This moves energy from crown to feet for grounding and increased energy. If I want to move energy from "earth to sky" (feet to head), all my crystal points will face the client's "north," or Crown Chakra. This moves the client's energy toward higher knowledge or spiritual experience. A trained healer will intuitively know in which direction to move energy.

7. Stones may be placed on one or many chakra points, and peppered around the perimeter of the client's body. I use my intuitive sight (I can see energy), my hands (I can feel energy), my feelings (I am empathic), and my intuition (I am claircognizant, which means I just know, without being able to explain how or why) to place the stones, or I'll use a pendulum to determine which chakras I will be working with in a session.

8. After the energy exchange has happened between the client and the stones, it is time to remove the stones. I use my shaman's rattle around the person's body to break up any dense energies and I brush off the client's body and aura with my feather fan and burn some sage. Then I ask the client to take a few very deep

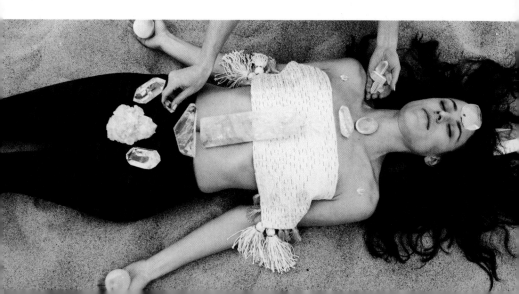

breaths to ground their energy, shake off any excess "energetic dust," and become present in the space again.

9. In order to close the "sacred space," I thank my Spirit Guides and my client's Spirit Guides for being present while facilitating the healing, and I close the Four Directions.

10. I help my client to sit up, give them some water, ask them how they are feeling, and invite them to share anything from the experience. I tell them to drink plenty of water after the session and to eat a salty or protein-based snack to help ground them. I also ask them to avoid alcohol for 24 hours before and 24 hours after a healing session.

11. When I am finished, I clean my crystals of any physical or energetic "dirt" and return my *khuyas* to my medicine bag or *mesa*.

Hot Tips

- The stone will let you know! A stone that is not needed for the session or is inappropriate for the client's energy will roll off their body or roll to another place where it is better utilized.
- If the receiver feels uncomfortable with a particular stone, remove it—its energy is not right for their needs.
- As a client's chakras and aura absorb the stone medicine and are balanced by the crystal energies, the stones may roll off. If a crystal does this during the healing, I do *not* put it back on the client's body.
- Crystals may be laid in geometric grids on and around the client. The body is the central point of the grid.
- This type of healing can be intense, and major energy shifts can happen. After a session, there may also be a physical detoxification process that can continue for up to a week. Journaling is a good way for the client to document the changes taking place.
- Smaller tumbled stones work best for stone healings. You can put them either directly on the skin or on top of fabric or clothing.

GET STONED ALONE: MY GREEN JUICE CHAKRA CLEANSE DELIVERED TO YOUR DOOR!

Below is a simple version of my Chakra Cleanse that you can do on your own at home once a week.

1. Find a quiet space where you won't be disturbed. Put your phone on airplane mode. This is a DO NOT DISTURB moment.

2. Open a "sacred space" around yourself. Think about creating a container of protection to hold your energy while you work.

3. Take a few deep breaths to get yourself into the "me time" zone. If you like candles, music, or diffused oils, add those to set the mood!

4. Ask yourself, *What do I need assistance with at the present moment?* and check in with your body. You may actually feel the answer in your body, in the form of a heaviness in your chest or a queasiness in your stomach. This is your body pointing to the chakra where you are holding on to an issue physically and energetically. If this feels too advanced or you don't trust yourself to figure out which chakra to focus on, refer to the explanation of the chakras on pages 38–43 to home in on which chakra is affected by your particular issue.

5. Once you have located the chakra you are working with, you are ready to place a corresponding crystal on that specific area. As a general rule of thumb, remember that the colors of crystals correspond to the chakra colors, so have an assortment of crystals to choose from before you begin.

6. Take deep, full, slow ocean breaths for 10 minutes. (I recommend setting a timer.) Ocean breaths are inspired by the sound and rhythm a wave has rolling gently up and back down a beach. It is a breath created when a person constricts the base of their

throat, controlling the movement of breath in and out of the body. Imagine that you are expelling whatever is bothering you from your body and into the stone. Next visualize light that is the color of the crystal resting on your body, or sparkly, diamond-quality white light entering the chakra.

7. End by closing your "sacred space." Basically, you are taking the lid off the container you created.

8. Burn sage with the door or window open to clear the area. Clean your crystal in any of the ways recommended in chapter 6.

9. Drink one full glass of water post-session.

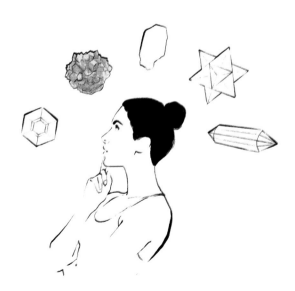

WHAT'S MY CRYSTAL RX?

I do a lot of custom prescriptions for my clients, and in this section, I'd like to share my top nine most requested formulas, so that you, too, can have them in your arsenal. If one of these prescriptions speaks to you, head over to StyleRituals.com to order one of my pre-cleansed and pre-charged Crystal Rx bags.

1. *The "Love It All" Bag:* To address all aspects of love, from calling in new relationships to dealing with heartbreak to working on loving yourself a little bit more.
   - Pink Botswana Agate
   - Rhodonite
   - Rose Quartz
   - Ruby Fuchsite
   - Watermelon Tourmaline

2. *The "I Mean Business" Bag:* Want to attract more money with a side dose of self-respect? This is your bag.
   - Bismuth
   - Black Obsidian
   - Citrine
   - Green Aventurine
   - Sardonyx
   - Sunstone

3. *The "Cosmic Cleaning Lady" Bag:* The A-game crystal gang for creating energetically clean spaces.
   - Amethyst
   - Black Kyanite
   - Selenite
   - Shungite
   - Smoky Quartz

4. *The "Chill the F*** Out" Bag:* Need to get off the hamster wheel? Here's your go-to.
   - Black Tourmaline
   - Dalmatian Stone
   - Lepidolite

5. *The "Speak Your Truth" Bag:* Do you solemnly swear that you will tell the truth, the whole truth, and nothing but the truth? Speak your personal truth with clarity, confidence, and continuity, while letting go of those outdated "cat got your tongue" traumas and dramas with this collection.
   - Blue Lace Agate
   - Blue Onyx
   - Lapis Lazuli
   - Sodalite

6. **The "Jet Setter" Bag:** This grouping helps you travel safe by staying "grounded," fighting jet lag, and sleeping through the baby crying three rows back.

   - Black Tourmaline
   - Hematite
   - Lepidolite
   - Tiger's Eye

7. **The "Go Big or Go Home" Bag:** A bag to help you manifest while honoring, living in the present, and being open to divine timing.

   - Charoite
   - Iron Pyrite
   - Titanium Quartz

8. **The "Study Buddy" Bag:** Need some extra clarity and insight while hitting the books? This grouping is your best study aid.

   - Blue Apatite
   - Danburite
   - Fluorite
   - Icelandic Spar (Optical Calcite)

9. **The "High Vibe" Bag:** Ready to level-up in the mystical realm? These are key crystals in any mystical girl's arsenal.

   - Aqua Aura Quartz
   - Astrophyllite
   - Blue Kyanite
   - Fairy Stone
   - Larvikite
   - Peacock Ore

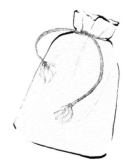

A LESSON IN COLOR PSYCHOLOGY

You may find you are repeatedly attracted to a certain crystal color, and that this crystal color may correspond to the colors you are naturally drawn to elsewhere in your life. For example, you walk into a crystal shop and notice that every stone you pick up, whether big, small, jagged, or smooth, is pink, the official color of bubble gum, cotton candy, and Barbie. What does this mean? Let's consult color psychology and our basic knowledge of the chakras for some insight into why we're attracted to certain colors.

CRYSTAL COLOR ENERGY GUIDE

The image at right, known as the Great Color Wheel of Life and Crystals, aligns each color with its meaning, as well as with a particular time of day and season. In contrast to astrological signs and other birthstone lists, the Great Color Wheel shows us the color that corresponds to our birth time and season, and it may explain why we are drawn to particular hues.

WINTER

Midwinter

20 Jan–18

Indi

Vi

T

Respect

Compass

Prophecy

Acceptanc

Recovery

Empathy

Practicality

Calmnes

Opennes

Flexibil

Spiri

19 Feb–19 Mar

Blue

Vernal Equinox

DAWN

20 Mar–19 Apr

Turquoise

SPRING

Mid-Spring

Apr–20 May

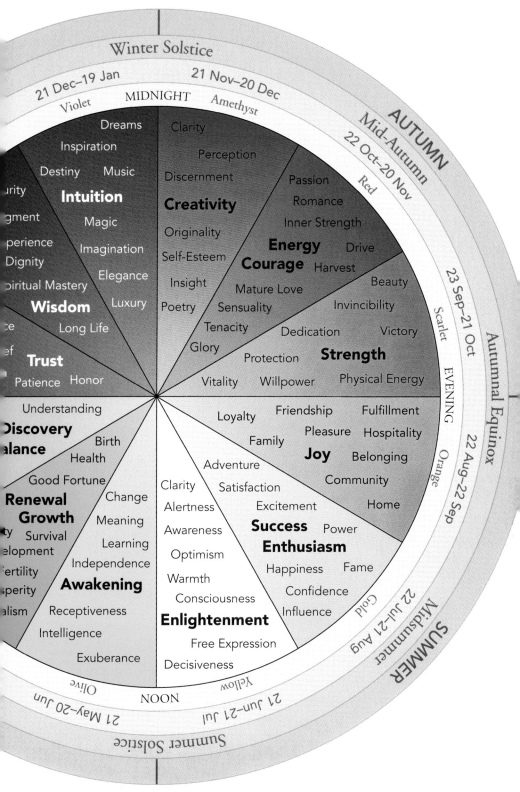

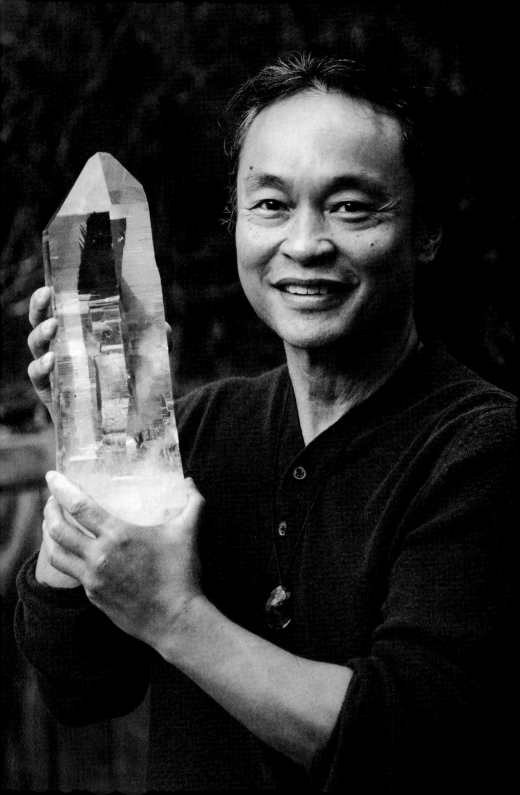

Who Taught Me About Stone Healing?

I AM TRULY BLESSED to have had many wise teachers on my crystal journey. Kirby Seid, a crystal expert based in the Bay Area, has been one of my key mentors. Kirby graduated from UC Santa Cruz with a degree in humanistic psychology, and then went on to start his gem and mineral business, Seid Crystals. He has been doing crystal consultations and light and sound healing with the help of crystals for thirty years, and he is a master stone carver who makes custom shamanic tools for teaching and healing practices. Kirby is truly a healer's healer, and a teacher's teacher.

Interview with Kirby Seid, Founder of Seid Crystals

How did you get into the crystal biz?

When I was a child, my dad worked for Shell oil. He would go to construction sites all over the world and bring me back fossils and crystals. Later in life, I wanted to start my own business. I looked at my crystal collection and thought it would allow me to travel the world. I started cutting crystals and became aware that certain things were happening around these crystals. There was an awakening in me; there was a quickening, if you will, as thought to manifestation was happening faster; I noticed the positive affect of them on myself and other people as I worked closer with them. I was wondering if I was doing damage to these life-forms by cutting them (into skulls, pyramids, faceted points, etc.), and who am I to decide what shape they should be? I was returning from my first trip getting crystals in Madagascar and stopped in Washington, D.C. That Monday morning, I sat on top of a huge quartz boulder at the Smithsonian and the crystals "let me know" that it was okay to cut them, and how to do it. They communicated to me that I just needed to get them into people's hands and that they wanted to work with the human kingdom. I got permission from the crystal and mineral kingdom to do this work. I also realized you don't just cut them willy-nilly—you look where the most power is coming from and cut accordingly.

Who taught you how to cut crystals?

Glen Spencer, a lapidary artist in Indianapolis, and Glen Laher, a famous carver, taught me how to cut crystals. Glen Laher taught me to be very precise with faceting.

Blow our minds and tell us something we don't know!

Let's talk about ways to clear a crystal that you may not know. Diamantina, or "Singing Crystals," will clear another crystal of any unwanted energy through sound. You can ping them like a tuning fork with a tiny metal mallet and its vibration will clear other crystals. Also, Marcel Vogel had a demagnetizer cleaner, and he would demagnetize crystals to make their energy "neutral, clear, or clean."

If you were a crystal, which crystal would you be?

Smoky Citrine Quartz

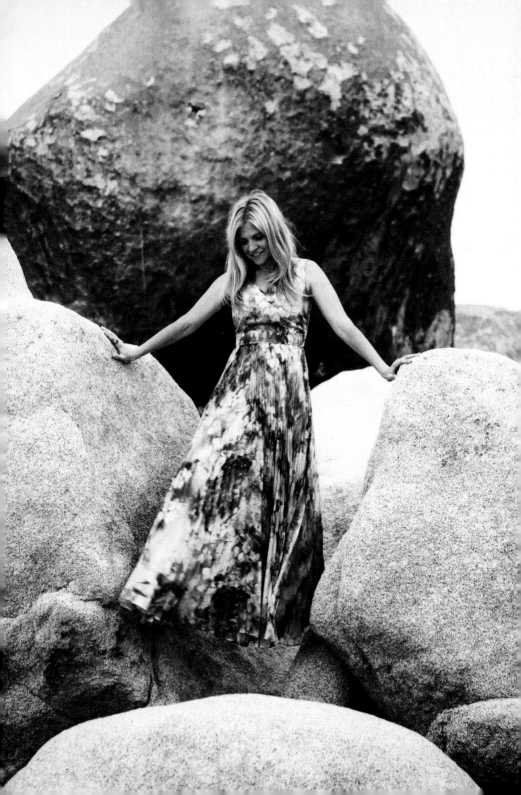

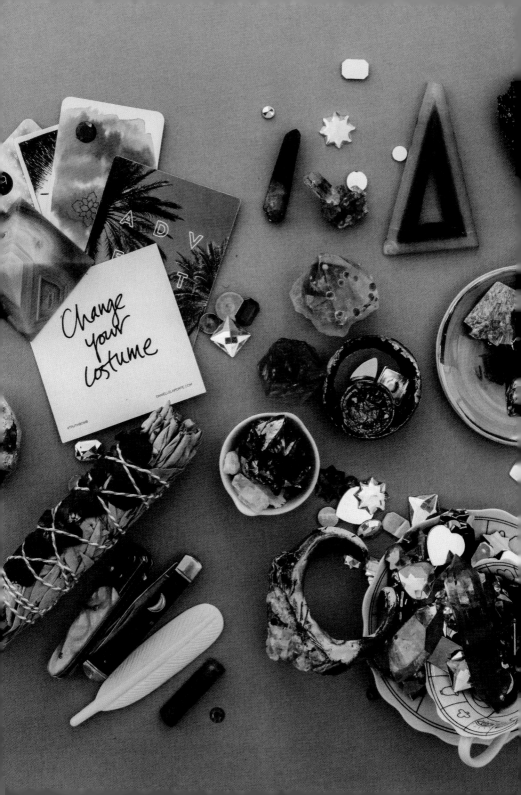

2

BUILDING YOUR CRYSTAL ARSENAL

The goal of a designer is to listen, observe, understand,
sympathize, empathize, synthesize, and glean insights that
enable him or her to make the invisible visible.

–HILLMAN CURTIS

THE TOP 20 STONES EVERY GIRL NEEDS IN HER ARSENAL

Building your crystal collection when you're just starting out can be
overwhelming, I know! Take a deep breath, and start small. These are
the twenty essential stones I would recommend for any beginner, based
on wisdom from my mentors and my own personal work with stones.
Each stone comes with a laundry list of mental, physical, spiritual, and
emotional benefits. I'll explain to you why each one is a must-have,
along with its corresponding "C Spot" (the chakra that it targets).

1. Amethyst

AKA: "The Vampire Slayer"

The Look: Deep purple

Where It Comes From: Argentina, Bolivia, Brazil, Canada, Russia, Siberia, South Korea, Sri Lanka, United States, Uruguay, Zambia

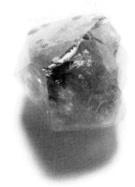

The "C Spot": 7th/Crown Chakra

Why You Need It in Your Life: When you want to "Just Say No!" Amethyst is used in crystal prescriptions for treating addiction, and addictions show up in our lives in all sorts of ways: alcohol, shoe shopping, negative self-talk, workaholism, smoking, social media, etc. Just about anything can become an addiction. Ever wonder why crystal stores always have a giant purple Amethyst geode in the corner of the room? It's because Amethyst rids a room of negative "energy vampires." It's also super high-vibration, and it helps us to tap into our intuition and to connect with higher planes of existence.

Mystical Homework: Make gem water by dropping a piece of tumbled Amethyst into your water, pitcher, water bottle, or drinking glass. Then drink the water! Make sure you clean your crystal, of course, before putting it into the water. As you hydrate, you'll be helping to curb bad habits. Amethyst water is absolutely safe to drink—some gem water is not—so please check a reliable source before doing this with other crystals.

Crystal Affirmation: "I am working on my personal addictions to the best of my abilities."

2. Black Obsidian

AKA: "Get Grounded"

The Look: Black, like your best go-to booties

Where It Comes From: Any place with high amounts of volcanic activity, including Argentina, Armenia, Azerbaijan, Australia, Canada, Chile, El Salvador, Georgia, Greece, Guatemala, Iceland, Italy, Japan, Kenya, Mexico, New Zealand, Papua New Guinea, Peru, Scotland, Turkey, United States

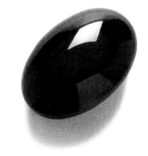

The "C Spot": 1st /Root Chakra

Why You Need It in Your Life: Obsidian rock forms when molten lava cools very quickly and forms into glass. It is associated with Pele, the Hawaiian goddess of fire. Its main uses are for grounding and protection, but Obsidian can also aid in past-life healing, sorting through misuses of power, calming a fiery temper, and releasing stuck emotions like fear, anger, stress, and resentment. Obsidian is a go-to stone for shamans, as it is highly protective when doing heavy-duty spiritual work.

Mystical Homework: Put Black Obsidian in your pillowcase or on your nightstand, or fall asleep with it in your hand to help decompress and ground yourself at the end of the day.

Crystal Affirmation: "I am one with the earth."

3. Bloodstone

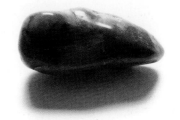

AKA: "Flex Your Muscles"

The Look: Hunter green with red freckles

Where It Comes From: Australia, Brazil, China, India, Madagascar, Scotland, United States

The "C Spot": 1st/Root Chakra

Why You Need It in Your Life:
Bloodstone is an ancient talisman of good health and long life. In Chinese medicine, blood and qi (also known as chi or prana, which is a person's "life force" or energy) have an inseparable relationship. Qi is said to command or move the blood through the body. Bloodstone is great for treating diabetes, blood disorders, and bad circulation; it's an immune system stimulator, fights inflammation and infection, promotes hormonal balance, boosts energy levels, and increases endurance in physical activity. Carry Bloodstone as a good-luck charm for sports competitions.

Mystical Homework: Keep Bloodstone by your side if you are starting a new exercise routine. Place Bloodstone topically on the related area to relieve varicose veins, reduce lower back pain, and relieve discomfort from mosquito bites.

Crystal Affirmation: "The force is strong."

4. Carnelian

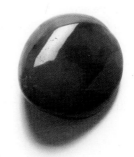

AKA: "So Emo"

The Look: Brownish red to orange

Where It Comes From: Brazil, Germany, India, Siberia, United States, Uruguay

The "C Spot": 2nd/Sacral Chakra

Why You Need It in Your Life: Carnelian is the stone of community and emotions, and it provides support for female reproductive issues, including easing period cramps and PMS, regulating menstrual cycles, and helping with infertility, fibroids, and uterine cysts.

Mystical Homework: Pack your Carnelian with your tampons! Menstruation is governed by the cycles of the moon, hence the phrase moon time. When you feel PMS symptoms coming, hold your Carnelian in your hand as much as you can. It is also helpful to lie down and put Carnelian on your abdomen during that time of the month.

Crystal Affirmation: "When emotions are high, intelligence is low." (Take a few deep breaths and wait for your emotions to settle before answering that email or text from the ex!)

5. Chrysocolla

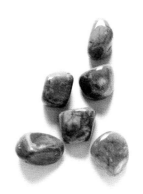

AKA: "Lady Power"

The Look: A mix of sky blue, blue, and blue-green

Where It Comes From: Chile, England, Israel, Mexico, Peru, Russia, United States, Zaire

The "C Spot": 4th/Heart Chakra

Why You Need It in Your Life: Also known as the Goddess Stone, Chrysocolla helps us to embrace the divine feminine through strong communication, self-expression, empowerment, and education. Chrysocolla stimulates the mind, and at the same time its calming effects allow our truth and inner wisdom to surface and be heard. This stone enhances the power that our words and actions have on those around us, and encourages compassion and strengthening of character. It also brings forth prosperity and eagle-eye discernment in business by sharpening our analytical and intuitive abilities. Chrysocolla is the stone of oracles, high priestesses, and medicine women everywhere; those drawn to it will feel a connection with ancient energies and indigenous wisdom traditions when they use it.

Mystical Homework: It's time to put your goddess voice to work! Let's raise our collective vibration by showing some love to other ladies out there. Every day for the next thirty days, make it a point to tell a woman in your life how much you respect who she is or what she does—or make a long overdue apology, if you need to. Once you have spoken to that woman (whether she's your mom, your best friend, a colleague, or a stranger), find a quiet place to sit and hold your crystal in your right hand (again, we send energy out of our right side). Visualize sending that woman some extra good vibes for a few minutes. According to universal law, what you put out will come back to you. So if you need a little love in your life, the best thing you can do is pre–pay it forward!

Crystal Affirmation: "I am worthy and deserving of giving and receiving love."

6. Citrine

AKA: "Work Your Mojo"

The Look: Golden yellow

Where It Comes From: Brazil, France, Madagascar, Russia

The "C Spot": 3rd/Solar Plexus Chakra

Why You Need It in Your Life: The stone of business and personal power, Citrine can catapult you into embracing a leadership role and making things happen in business. This gemstone is

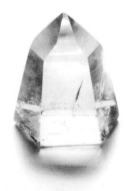

associated with creativity and wealth. Not only can Citrine help you with, say, asking for and getting a long overdue raise, it can help you to stand firmly within your personal power and self-confidence, and establish healthy boundaries, in every area of your life.

Mystical Homework: Create a thirty-day Abundance Altar with the "Merchant's Stone"! Place your piece of Citrine on top of a stack of clean, crisp $1 bills on your desk. (I do this with one hundred $1 bills, but use the number of bills that feel right or are symbolic to you.) The new bills are meant to symbolize the fresh energy of the money that you want to have coming in. In addition to the Citrine, add other items that symbolize power and abundance for you to your altar. These could be things like a small statue of Lakshmi (the Hindu goddess of wealth and prosperity) or a picture of someone you really admire in business. In the Chinese Buddhist fêng shui tradition, you could also add a small "money tree" to your altar (basically, any small green tree or plant), as the green leaves represent money, prosperity, and growth. Once you've decorated your Abundance Altar, burn some sage or palo santo to clear the surrounding air, and then spend some time in front of your altar visualizing what you would like to call into your life, money- and success-wise. You can also hold the money and Citrine in your hands as you visualize. Repeat this ritual once a day for thirty days.

Crystal Affirmation: "I am abundant."

7. Clear Quartz

AKA: "Black Skinny Jeans"
The Look: Clear. Colorless. Transparent.
Where It Comes From: Brazil, Canada, China, Germany, Madagascar, Peru, South Africa, United States

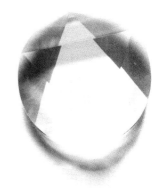

The "C Spot": Targets all the chakras, but especially the 7th/Crown Chakra

Why You Need It in Your Life: Clear Quartz is a wardrobe staple, like your black skinny jeans. It goes with all your other crystals, and it's not only a neutral, it's an amplifier. Clear Quartz is known as the "Master Healer" and "High Channeler," and you can pair it with any other crystal to amplify what that other crystal does. It's used for connecting with your higher self, your intuition, and your Spirit Guides.

Mystical Homework: Try a one-week meditation practice. On day one, hold your Clear Quartz in your left hand (energy comes in through the left hand, on the divine feminine side of the body), and pick seven other stones—one for each day of the week—to hold in your right hand (the divine masculine side of your body). By holding the stones, you are getting to know them and activating them. Close your eyes, get still, and breathe deeply for 10 minutes, visualizing what each individual crystal in your right hand can help you to accomplish in your life. Then, for each of the next seven days, pick one of your seven crystals and repeat this practice while holding the colored stone in your right hand and the Clear Quartz in your left hand. The Clear Quartz will amplify the powers of the other stone you are holding that day. Just don't forget to breathe!

Crystal Affirmation: "I am a clear and present channel of divine light and love."

8. Garnet

AKA: "The Magnum"

The Look: Dark red, like your favorite fall nail polish

Where It Comes From: Brazil, Canada, China, Czech Republic, Finland, India,

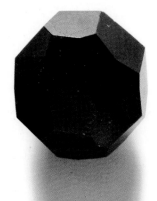

Kenya, Madagascar, Myanmar, Namibia, Norway, South Africa, Sri Lanka, Tanzania, Thailand, United States, Zambia

The "C Spot": 4th/Heart Chakra

Why You Need It in Your Life: This is the ultimate "life force" stone. A little history: The name "garnet" comes from the Latin word *garanatus,* meaning "seedlike," which refers to the small, bright red seeds of the pomegranate. The use of red Garnet in ancient ritual dates back thousands of years to the Egyptian pharaohs and the ancient Romans. The Garnet is a stone of health; it energizes, balances, reduces toxins, strengthens, purifies vital organs and blood, and promotes absorption of vitamins and minerals within the body. Not to mention that as a heart-based stone, it inspires love, devotion, and passion between the sheets. Garnet is referred to throughout the Bible by the alternate name "carbuncle," and all sorts of myths have been attached to the stone. One of the most memorable is the medieval belief that a dragon's eyes were made of Garnet. In the Far East, Garnet was believed to stanch the flow of blood and to have the ability to inflict mortal wounds when fired out of guns or thrown with a slingshot.

Mystical Homework: Meditate with a Garnet on your chest to revitalize the body and get your blood flowing!

Crystal Affirmation: "I am full of energy."

9. Iron Pyrite

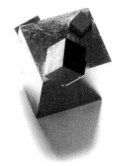

AKA: "The World is Your Oyster"

The Look: Shiny, gold

Where It Comes From: Australia, France, Germany, Italy, Peru, Russia, Taiwan, United States

The "C Spot": 3rd/Solar Plexus Chakra

Why You Need It in Your Life: Pyrite is called "Fool's Gold" because it resembles gold to the untrained eye, but there is nothing foolish about this manifesting powerhouse. "Pyrite" comes from the Greek word *pyr*, meaning "fire," because sparks fly from it when it is hit with another mineral or metal. Traditionally known to generate wealth, Pyrite carries a super-masculine vibe, and it's great when we want to channel our divine masculine for confidence, willpower, persistence, and getting things done! The design junkie in me loves this stone big time, because it naturally grows in perfectly formed squares.

Mystical Homework: On the first day of a new moon (the best day of the month to call in what you want in life), write a "Manifestation List" of important things you want to accomplish. Place your Iron Pyrite on top of your written list, and reread and reflect on the list every day to help the items on it manifest. Remember: Our thoughts reflect our present reality, so take this part seriously. Let it all marinate until the next full moon, and then burn or "release" the list so the universe can do its work from there.

Crystal Affirmation: "I create my own reality."

10. Labradorite

AKA: "The Magic Maker"

The Look: Iridescent blue green . . . like peacock feathers

Where It Comes From: Canada, Finland, Mexico, Madagascar, Newfoundland, Norway, South America, United States

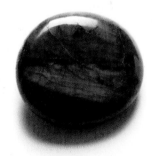

The "C Spot": 6th/Third-Eye Chakra

Why You Need It in Your Life: Yes, it's as enchanting as it looks! If you want to create a closer relationship with your mystical side, call on the "Stone of Magic." According to ancient legend, the Inuit people believed Labradorite was formed by the northern lights, or aurora borealis, that shone down on the shores of Labrador in Canada. "Labradorescence" was captured inside the rocks on the shore, resulting in the fiery reflection that appears on this stone's surface. It awakens our psychic abilities, feeds our imagination, opens our wisdom channels, stimulates transformation, and brings out one's adventurous side, which you will definitely need when jumping down any mystical rabbit hole. Labradorite is a must-have fave of healers worldwide.

Mystical Homework: Attend a Moon Ceremony, and take your new pet rock with you. Place it on the altar at the center of the Moon Circle for the duration of the ceremony so it can energetically soak up the high vibes.

Crystal Affirmation: "I cultivate my own magic."

11. Lapis Lazuli

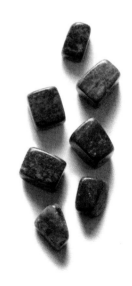

AKA: "Full Communicado"

The Look: Deep, royal blue

Where It Comes From: Afghanistan, Canada, Chile, India, Italy, Madagascar, Mongolia, Pakistan, Russia, United States, Uruguay

The "C Spot": 5th/Throat Chakra

Why You Need It in Your Life: Lapis Lazuli is the "Stone of Communication." It promotes speaking one's truth with grace and confidence, and it eases communication issues and breakdowns.

Mystical Homework: Place Lapis Lazuli on your throat while you meditate, and envision yourself in a difficult conversation, speaking your truth. Imagine being open to hearing both sides of the conversation while respectfully and lovingly speaking your truth. Deathly afraid of public speaking? Use Lapis Lazuli as your worry stone: Hold it in your hand when rehearsing your speech, as well as when it's time to step up to the mic on the day of your speech. Let the stone absorb your anxieties.

Crystal Affirmation: "I will speak my truth with clarity and confidence."

12. Lepidolite

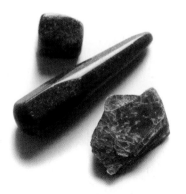

AKA: "Crystal Xanax"

The Look: Purple with a hint of white spotting, like freckles

Where It Comes From: Brazil, Canada, Madagascar, Russia, United States

The "C Spot": 4th/Heart Chakra

Why You Need It in Your Life: Who doesn't need to chill the f*** out?

Mystical Homework: Place it by your bedside to help you sleep, or use it to meditate and relax.

Crystal Affirmation: "I am calm, dammit. I swear!"

13. Malachite

AKA: "Better Than Botox"

The Look: Green

Where It Comes From: Australia, Chile, Germany, Mexico, South Africa, Romania, Russia, United States, Zaire

The "C Spot": 4th/Heart Chakra

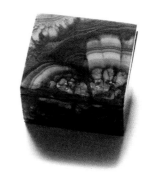

Why You Need It in Your Life: If it was good enough for Cleopatra, then it's good enough for me! Ancient Egyptians used Malachite in eyeliner, and it was used in the Eye of Horus symbol (for protection, royal power, and good health) on Egyptian temples. Malachite absorbs energy and draws emotions to the surface, and it promotes physical and emotional healing by drawing out impurities . . . making it a fave in the beauty industry. Known as the "Stone of the Midwife," Malachite works with female-centric issues, like regulating the menstrual cycle, cramps, sexual trauma, and easing labor. Believed to be a "Stone of Transformation," it assists with transitions and facilitates spiritual growth. P.S. For all you jet-setters out there, it alleviates fears of flying and travel sickness.

Mystical Homework: Put it on your face! Rich in copper, Malachite's anti–free radical properties help to protect cellular structures, and it works as a skin-conditioning agent, combating daily stresses and acting as an after-sun ingredient. I recommend Tracie Martyn Complexion Savior, a skincare mask that contains Malachite.

Crystal Affirmation: "I am flaw-some."

14. Nirvana Quartz (Himalayan Ice Quartz)

AKA: "Inner Focus"

The Look: Pale, translucent pink or colorless. It looks like a mini iceberg.

Where It Comes From: The Himalayan Mountain Range

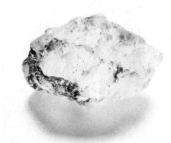

The "C Spot": 6th/Third-Eye Chakra and 7th/Crown Chakra

Why You Need It in Your Life: This is a newer crystal, as it was discovered in 2006 when the glaciers in the Himalayan mountain range began to melt and recede. It's estimated that this variety of quartz had lain under those glaciers for thousands of years before being discovered, and it isn't found anywhere else on Earth. Nirvana or Himalayan Ice Quartz promotes an inner focus and peace, and it's perfect for holding during meditation practices.

Mystical Homework: Can't sit still? I get it. Put your phone on airplane mode and meditate with your Nirvana Quartz. Start with 5 minutes a day, then build up to 10 minutes, then 20. It's like exercise: You need to build your stamina. For help with focus, and instruction on technique, enroll in a meditation course, or else there are some great meditation apps out there that can help. My picks for beginners are Headspace, 10% Happier, and OMG. I Can Meditate!

Crystal Affirmation: "Nothing rocks me."

15. Rose Quartz

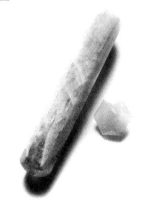

AKA: "The Love Doctor"

The Look: Light pink

Where It Comes From: Brazil, Germany, India, Madagascar, United States

The "C Spot": 4th/Heart Chakra

Why You Need It in Your Life: Rose Quartz activates the heart chakra and enhances all types of love: self-love, unconditional love, and love for others. This baby-pink stone is no softie as it raises self-esteem; promotes positive energy; restores confidence; helps with emotional balance; releases stress, tension, and anger; and helps curb jealousy.

Mystical Homework: Make your own "Love Mist" spray with rose quartz. First, clean your Rose Quartz crystal using sage, sunlight, moonlight, or salt water. Place your Rose Quartz in a glass bowl of filtered water in direct sunlight, and leave it there until sundown. Then pour the crystal-charged water into a glass mister bottle, and add 22 drops of argan oil (jojoba and almond oil also work well) and 11 drops of rose oil. Give it a shake and mist yourself whenever you feel like you need a little pick-me-up in the love department. In addition to the positive vibes of Rose Quartz, you'll also benefit from the rose oil, which is super good for your skin: It's antimicrobial, combats acne, reduces inflammation and redness, tones and tightens skin, fades scars, and refines skin texture.

Crystal Affirmation: "The biggest show of love I can give is by loving myself, first and foremost."

16. Selenite

AKA: "The Cosmic Colonic"

The Look: Shiny and milky white

Where It Comes From: Australia, England, France, Germany, Greece, Mexico, Peru, Poland, United States

The "C Spot": 7th/Crown Chakra

Why You Need It in Your Life: Use Selenite to cleanse your closet and your aura! This crystal wonder clears the stuck, dense, unwanted energy out of your personal space. Use a big piece of Selenite like a metal detector and wave it over the front and back of your body to clear out all the smog that has accumulated in your energy field and in your physical body. This crystal is self-cleaning, so you never need to give it a bath. Selenite is named after the Greek goddess of the moon, Selene; it increases libido and promotes fertility, inner peace, and clarity. It's also great for meditation and for contacting your Spirit Guides.

Mystical Homework: Place Selenite in areas where energy tends to get stuck, like doorways, window ledges, under the bed, in the four corners of a room, and most definitely in your closet!

Crystal Affirmation: "I release anything that does not belong to me."

17. Shungite

AKA: "The Technology Cleanse"

The Look: Matte or shiny black

Where It Comes From: Deposits near Shunga village, in Karelia, Russia

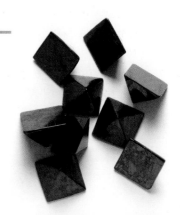

The "C Spot": 1st/Root Chakra

Why You Need It in Your Life: Protection from *man-made* electromagnetic frequencies (EMFs), which are invisible waves that emanate from any electrical device. Low-frequency EMFs are emitted from appliances and electronics, and high-frequency EMFs originate from wireless devices. Our bodies also have a natural EMF system; when man-made EMFs enter our energy field it can throw us out of whack and cause what's known as subliminal stress to our systems.

Mystical Homework: Keep Shungite close to all your electronic devices, including your computer, iPad, TV, cell phone, microwave, and fuse box. You can even get little sticky-backed low-profile pieces of Shungite to put on the outside of your cell phone.

Crystal Affirmation: "I am protected."

18. Smoky Quartz

AKA: "The Designated Driver"

The Look: Translucent brownish gray

Where It Comes From: Australia, Brazil, Madagascar, Mozambique, Scotland, Switzerland, United States

The "C Spot": 1st/Root Chakra

Why You Need It in Your Life: Negative thoughts and actions, be gone! In ancient times, Druids used Smoky Quartz as a Stone of Power, and today, we work with it as an amulet of protection. Smoky Quartz helps guard your home and possessions from damage, theft, and accidents. This stone absorbs negative energy, and relieves tension, stress, and anxiety. It also energetically removes toxins from the adrenal glands, kidneys, and pancreas.

Mystical Homework: Keep Smoky Quartz in your car, as it can help with road rage and protect you from accidents while driving!

Crystal Affirmation: "I will not succumb to negative thoughts or actions. Life is too short. I will let it go."

19. Sunstone

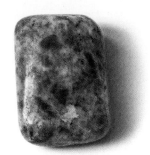

AKA: "Make It or Break It"

The Look: '80s salmon pink (like your grandma's house in Florida)

Where It Comes From: Norway, Siberia, Sweden, United States

The "C Spot": 1st/Root Chakra

Why You Need It in Your Life: Known as the "Stone of Career and Leadership," this workplace crystal can bring about opportunities for personal promotion and help you establish boundaries against situations that could potentially drain your finances.

Mystical Homework: Trying to stake out a new career path? It's vision board time. Pull photos, magazine clips, and other bits of career inspo and piece them all together on your vision board. Then place your Sunstone on top and let things cook. When putting together a vision board, either on paper or on Pinterest, keep in mind that it's time to think BIG! Ask yourself, *What is the best that could happen?* Close your eyes and tap into what those big dreams look, feel, taste, and smell like.

Crystal Affirmation: "I am successful at whatever I put my mind to."

20. Yellow Tiger's Eye

AKA: "The Travel Junkie"

The Look: Streaked brown and yellow, resembling a cat's eye

Where It Comes From: Australia, Brazil, China, India, Myanmar, South Africa, Spain, United States

The "C Spot": 3rd/Solar Plexus Chakra

Why You Need It in Your Life: Rawr! Tiger's Eye is an ancient talisman, known as the "all-seeing, all-knowing eye." Ancients believed that Tiger's Eye granted its wearer the ability

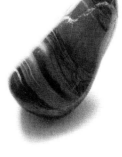

to observe everything around them, and it is also known as an ancient "gazing" stone, used by female shamans to provide powers of the "far-seeing eye." Ancient Roman soldiers are also said to have carried it for protection in battle. Today it is associated with courage, integrity, protecting one's resources, deflecting malignity, rational decision-making, quick thinking, and sharp inner vision. And my personal favorite: It is *the* stone for protection during travel.

Mystical Homework: Trains, planes, and automobiles . . . Keep Tiger's Eye in your carry-on, and ask for protection from your Spirit Guides before you set out on an adventure.

Crystal Affirmation: "I am safe no matter where I roam."

CRYSTAL SILHOUETTES: THE 11 BASIC SHAPES AND THEIR USES

Crystals have unique uses, and they excel at different tasks depending on their shape. These are the most common, practical, and adored silhouettes that I recommend for beginners (although there are many more):

1. **Ball or Sphere:** This shape emits and evenly distributes energy through a space, making it great to hold in meditation. If you really want to go for it, you can also use this shape for what is known as "crystal gazing" or "scrying." Scrying is the art of looking into a reflective surface, such as water, glass, mirror, or crystal, to gain mystical insight, and it has been practiced with crystal balls for thousands of years. Mystics believe you can get a glimpse into the past, present, or future with this technique.

2. **Cluster:** A group of crystals growing together from one base. Clusters radiate energy out into every direction equally (like light from a disco ball), and they work well for directing and cleansing the energy in a room. Great for home, office, or your sacred space.

3. **Single Terminated Point:** These can occur naturally, but they are also sometimes cut to a point by lapidaries. Single terminated point crystals are useful for directing energy toward a specific intention or purpose (think of a finger pointing at something). Great for beginners, and commonly used in crystal gridding.

4. **Double Terminated Point:** These crystals are pointy or terminated on both ends, and they can emit and receive energy in both directions. They transfer energy back and forth—like a text convo—and are useful for moving energy between two places, people, or ideas. They promote alignment, balance, and healing,

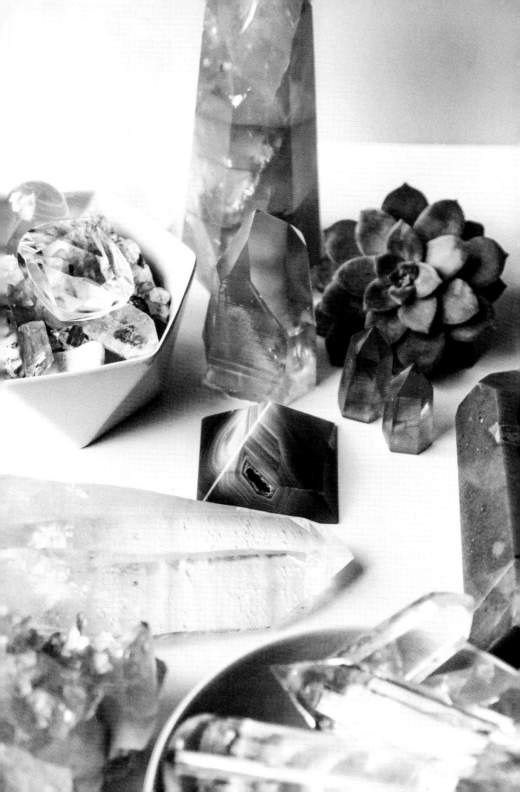

and can also direct energy between two chakras of the body. For example, if you have been feeling like your heart is saying one thing, while something else is flying out of your mouth, lay the crystal between your 4th and 5th chakras to get them to communicate better.

5. *Egg:* Egg-shaped crystals can detect energy imbalances within the body and rebalance these blockages. They are ideal for meditation practices, and the more pointed end of the egg is useful as a reflexology or acupressure tool.

6. *Geode:* Geodes are an example of how you can never judge a book by its cover. They're rough and ugly on the outside, but when cracked open, they reveal a twinkling inner cavity lined with crystals. Due to their rounded, cavelike shape, they can hold energy like a storage container and then amplify and release this energy in a slow and steady manner, like a room diffuser. Geodes are useful for protection, aid in spiritual growth, and assist in breaking addictions.

7. *Cube or Square:* These shapes consolidate energy and are useful for anchoring intention and for grounding. Naturally occurring square crystals, like Fluorite or Iron Pyrite, can draw off negative energy and transform it into positive.

8. *Heart:* No surprise here, heart-shaped crystals attract loving energy. They're also great for dealing with the tough stuff: sadness, grief, suffering, breakups, losses, pain. Rumor has it that this shape also increases fertility.

9. *Twin Crystal (aka Soul Mate Crystal):* A twin crystal is two crystals that have grown together and are attached side by side to a common base. These promote communication and togetherness. An excellent crystal for working on relationships.

10. *Pyramid:* Let's travel back to ancient Egypt! The Great Pyramids were believed to be structures that gathered spiritual energy through their points. Pyramid-shaped crystals do something similar, directing positive energy upward to increase psychic connection and relieving blockages in the chakras.

11. *The Magic Wand:* Crystal wands have no pointed end, but rather two rounded ends, with one side being wider, and they are helpful for moving energy. Wands are traditional healing tools for all types of healers, but they're especially popular with massage therapists and reflexologists.

WHAT'S THE DEAL WITH CRYSTAL SKULLS?

Crystal skulls are common in the gem world, carved from large pieces of crystal by a lapidary (an artisan who cuts or polishes gemstones) into a shape that resembles the human skull, and they date back to ancient times. The energy of a piece of crystal changes when it is carved into a particular shape (as noted above, different shapes are used for different work), so let's explore what skulls exude. In my experience, I've found that people are either *very* drawn to skulls, or totally turned off by them. It is believed that crystal skulls are "ancient computers" (meaning a powerful receptacle for stored information that can aid in healing, transmit energy, and have strong positive effects on one's spiritual growth), and that they contain messages, healing properties, and teachings from the universe that can help us advance both individually and collectively. Historically, Clear Quartz is the stone most commonly associated with crystal skulls, along with Amethyst, Golden Healer, Hematite, Lapis Lazuli, Rose Quartz, and Obsidian.

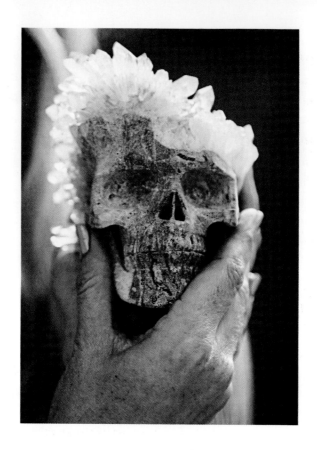

HOW TO USE CRYSTAL SKULLS ON THE DAILY

The best way to work with crystal skulls is to use them much like our ancestors did: Simply meditate while holding the skull. If you want to step it up and get mystical, try the ancient art of scrying: staring at your crystal with intention in a deep state of relaxation. Here's how it's done:

1. Sit face-to-face with your skull.
2. Take a few deep yoga-style breaths, clear your mind as best you can, and relax your eyes (if your vision blurs a bit, that's A-OK).

3. Align your eyes with the eye area of the skull.
4. Put forth a particular intention or question.
5. At this point, everyone's experience varies. You may see, hear, feel, or experience a response or sense of knowing around the intentions you created or the questions you asked.

PROPHECY OF THE 13 SKULLS

This one is straight out of Indiana Jones. Legend states that thirteen life-size master crystal skulls were scattered across the earth by a mysterious ancient society. These skulls are thought to be great houses of knowledge, containing information about this ancient society, the history of our planet, our purpose here on Earth, and the keys for unlocking all the great mysteries of the universe. (*All that contained in a few crystals?* I know.) According to legend, at some point in the future when our civilization is at a crossroads, all thirteen crystal skulls will be discovered and reunited, and their secrets will be unlocked, allowing human consciousness to evolve. Where are they now? Rumor has it that some are being safeguarded by shamans in remote locations, while others remain in the hands of those who are not yet aware of their importance.

CURATING YOUR SACRED CRYSTAL SPACE

Once you've collected your crystal essentials based on this list, your next task is to create a sacred space for your crystal practice. You can draw design inspiration for your space from holy places or sanctuaries that speak to you—temples, mosques, cathedrals, gardens, art museums, or even your favorite boutique. Remember, anywhere can be a sanctuary as long as it has meaning to you. Choose a location that suits your needs, and make it yours, whether it's a space in your bedroom, your home library, your garden or backyard, or on your fire escape.

This should be a very personal place where you can go to silence your mind, give thanks for what you have, reflect on what you want to invite into your life, and honor the things and the people you love.

Once you've decided on a space, it's time for some personal curation. In addition to crystals, add pictures of loved ones, tarot cards, flowers, statues, vision boards, jewelry, fabric, candles, and any other items that are meaningful to you, or that inspire on a mental, physical, emotional, or spiritual/energetic level.

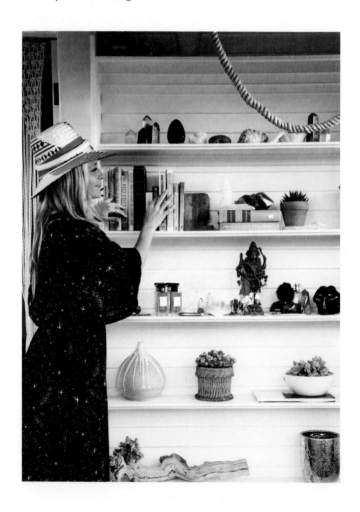

WHERE ELSE ARE CRYSTALS USED? EVERYWHERE!

Aside from your carefully chosen sacred space, there are plenty of other useful places for crystals in your abode, including:

1. *Your closet:* Closets hold our past, present, and what we are trying to manifest in the future. So shake out those energetic cobwebs and moths! Keep Selenite in your closet to clear the dense energy, or put a piece in the pocket of your favorite blazer to clear away the bad vibes from a sh*tty meeting with your boss!

2. *Under the bed:* Put Black Tourmaline under your bed for grounding and protection.

3. *On your nightstand:* Put dream crystals like Danburite, Herkimer Diamond, or Dream Quartz on your nightstand for restful sleep or for better dream recall.

4. *At work:* Make your desk at work your personal mission-control command center. Crystals like Amethyst or Citrine in your workspace will keep away toxic co-workers and call more business success into your life.

5. *In your handbag:* Where are my keys, not to mention my sanity? Who hasn't looked into that silk-lined abyss and thought, *If only I could get my purse organized, I could get the rest of my life in check*? Dumortierite enhances organizational skills, in addition to promoting peace, tranquility, and patience as we move through our hectic day-to-day lives.

6. *In your bra:* I consider this a second purse! Drop some Rose Quartz into your Agent Provocateur for a little extra self-love, and for that push (or push-up?) to show a little more love to others.

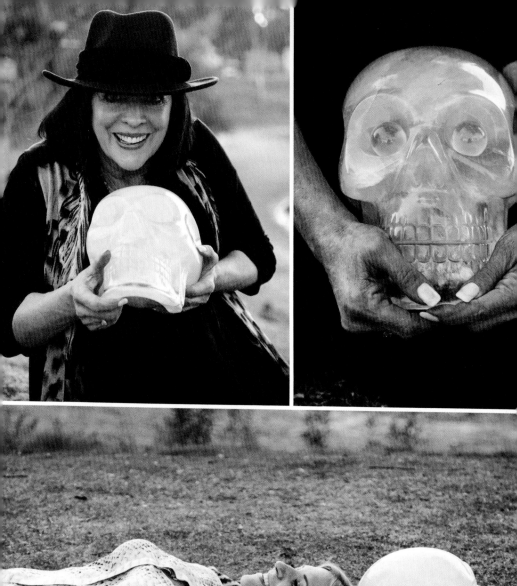
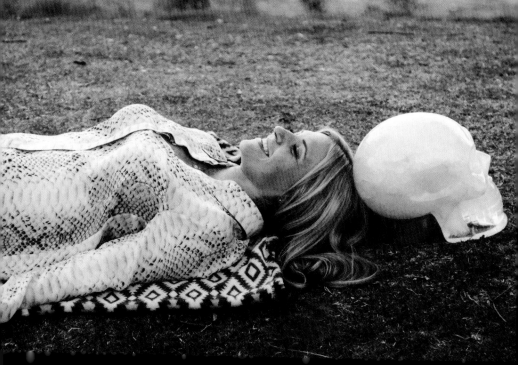

Interview with Carolyn Ford and "Einstein, the Skull of Consciousness"

CAROLYN IS A FRIEND AND FELLOW HEALER who also originally comes from the fashion world. She works with an incredibly powerful, seventy-thousand-year-old, thirty-three-pound ancient crystal skull named Einstein. Yes, you heard me correctly! My private one-hour activation session with Carolyn began with her examining my "Human Design" chart, followed by words of wisdom on behalf of Einstein, and then twenty minutes of meditation with my hands resting on Einstein. Read on for more!

How did you become the guardian of Einstein?

In 1989, I experienced a dream workshop with a medicine man who offered meditation with a contemporary carved crystal skull. I had never seen one before. He handed me a little carved crystal skull to hold during meditation and I immediately started to feel a connection with it. I meditated with the skull and asked if it had a message for me. The skull spoke to me and said, "You are the guardian."

I didn't know what that meant, but I knew that I needed to start working with a crystal skull, so I began looking for one of my own. I called some friends in Seattle who owned a crystal store and asked if they could help me find the right one. My friends called back to say they had found my skull, but that I would have to fly to Seattle to get it because it was a little bit bigger than anticipated. I expected a little 2- or 3-inch skull. Instead, I received Einstein.

What is Einstein?

He is the largest and most anatomically correct ancient crystal skull in the world. Einstein is considered an "ancient computer." In German *Ein* means "one" and *Stein* means "stone." Einstein was discovered by an explorer in the 1920s or '30s and brought back to be a part of the man's vast collection.

How much does Einstein weigh?

Thirty-three pounds.

How old is Einstein, and how long have you two been working together?

Einstein is approximately seventy thousand years old, and we've been working together since 1990.

Who carved Einstein?

He wasn't carved, he was created.

What do you and Einstein do?

We tour the world teaching people about crystal medicine and working with crystal skulls. At our public speaking engagements, I tell my story of meeting Einstein, and I communicate messages I receive from Einstein to the attendees. In private sessions, Einstein and I work with a technique brought to me by the man who had the revelation, Ra Uru Hu. It is called "The Human Design System." This is a revealed science that illustrates the mechanics of who you are based on your genetic blueprint. We want to help people realize their potential, upgrade their personal infrastructure, and align with their true nature.

Where did you receive your metaphysical training?

I studied with Hawaiian kahunas, Native American elders, Peruvian shamans, and an East Indian guru.

If you were a crystal, which one would you be?

Clear Quartz

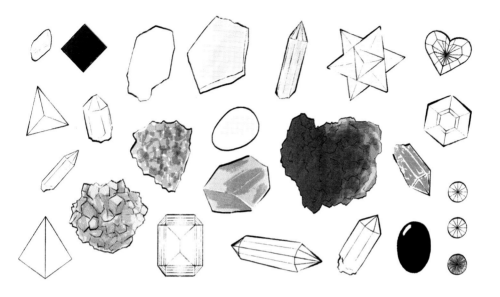

CRYSTAL PAIRINGS

Are there certain crystals that absolutely should or shouldn't be used together? The answer is yes. When working with two or more stones at the same time, you want them to harmonize. The key is to choose crystals that will work well together toward a common goal, rather than getting their energetic signals crossed. The last thing you want to create is crystal chaos.

Anyone can make or design their own crystal pairings. All you have to do is ask yourself what you are trying to achieve with your crystal blend and then identify the crystals whose qualities match your needs. For example: If you are trying to relax, meditate, or get to sleep, you don't want to hold a stone like Carnelian, which embodies vibrant, fiery energy. Instead, pick a crystal like Scolecite that promotes restful vibes. It's a bit like picking face products based on your skin type.

Here are some examples of a few crystal pairings, some harmonious and some not:

Dalmatian Stone + Dream Quartz =
ZZZzzzzzzzzzzzzzzz

Dalmatian Stone (yes, it's a white- to cream-colored stone with spots!) helps you to get off the hamster wheel of life and slow down. Dream Quartz does exactly what you would think, given its name. Together, these stones will help you to sleep better, and to be more calm and better rested when you wake up.

Blue Lace Agate + Carnelian =
Oil and Water

Blue Lace Agate helps to calm one's energy, whereas Carnelian carries a lot of fire and activity. The energies cancel each other out, so *do not* use them together.

Moldavite + Jet =
High-Vibe Meditation

Moldavite is a super-high-vibe meteorite that lets you explore the depth of the cosmos. But as my teacher Marcela Lobos would always say, "The more grounded you are, the farther out you can go. The stronger your tether or kite string, the higher you can fly." Jet, on the other hand, is great for grounding, as well as attracting knowledge and wisdom. This combo is perfect for a full-on esoteric meditation session.

Amethyst + Hematite =
Just Say NO

Dr. Mona Dinari, a brilliant Daoist acupuncturist who uses crystals in her treatments (and who we'll hear more from later in the book) told me that this is an inauspicious combination. Hematite carries the most "gravity" or weight of any crystal, and Amethyst is a "water" stone. And when you mix weight and water, you know what you get? Bloating! Avoid this combo.

Now that you've got the basics on how to build your crystal arsenal, how various crystal types and shapes converse with one another, and how you can create your own sacred space for your crystal practice, let's move on to what I like to call #ancientfuture. Here we will discuss the many fascinating ways in which crystals are used, and how scientists and mystics may actually be able to meet in the middle on this whole crystal convo.

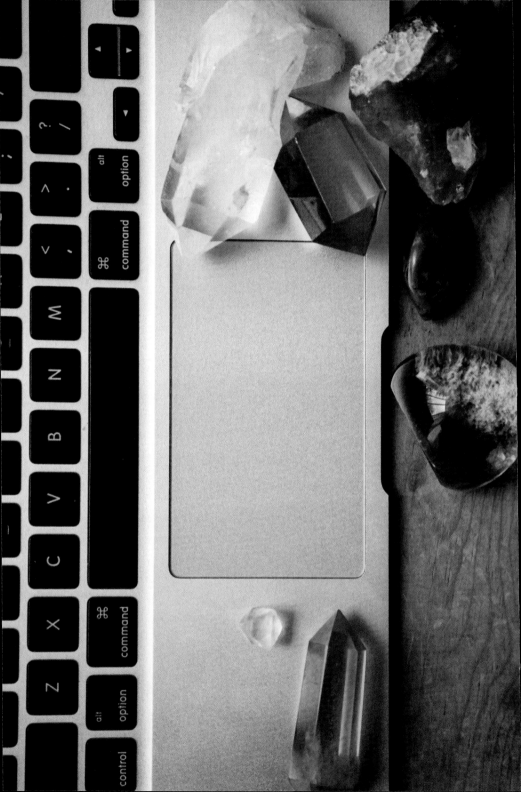

3

CRYSTAL INTELLIGENCE

What Does Science Have to Say?

In a crystal we have clear evidence of the existence
of a formative life-principle, and though we cannot
understand the life of a crystal, it is none the
less a living being.

—NIKOLA TESLA

LONG BEFORE PRESCRIPTION DRUGS, hospitals, and talk therapy existed, our ancestors turned to stones and crystals to recalibrate energy in the body, as preventative medicine, and to heal on a mental, physical, emotional, or spiritual/energetic level. Ancient babe-bosses wore crystals for knowledge, protection, healing, personal power, guidance, creativity, and connection. The Sumerians are the first early society known to use crystals for healing purposes, as far back as 4000 BC. Let's talk about who wore what, and who wore it best, in the cradles of civilization.

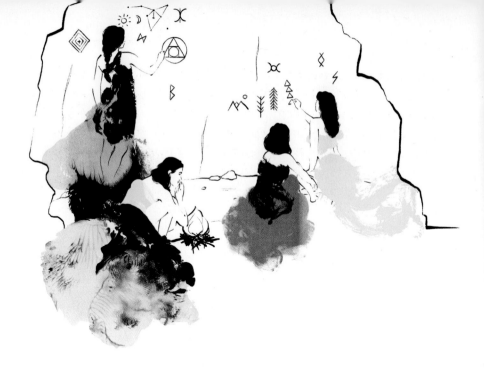

EGYPT

Cleopatra never left home without her wig or her Malachite eyeliner! The ancient Egyptians were big proponents of healing crystals, and Queen Cleopatra actually had an arsenal of crystal cosmetics on her vanity. She used bright green Malachite paste to line her lower lids, and a blend of shiny gold Iron Pyrite and electric blue Lapis Lazuli on her upper eyelids. Cleo and her crew wore makeup made of Lapis Lazuli to honor the goddess Isis and to promote enlightenment. But Cleo wasn't all flash. She also started the very practical trend of wearing black kohl pigment around the eye to protect from the bright midday sun. Ancient Egyptians were also equal makeup opportunists. Both men and women were known to wear copious amounts of gem-tastic makeup, which they believed conjured up the protection of the gods Horus and Ra as well as being antibacterial and warding off illnesses.

Crystal love in ancient Egypt didn't stop there. The Egyptians buried their dead with quartz on the forehead to help guide the departed safely to the afterlife. Pharaohs and priests also carried cylinders filled with quartz to balance energies within the body. Dancing girls and ladies of the night in ancient Egypt wore rubies in their belly buttons to increase their sex appeal. The Egyptians wore crystals over their hearts to attract love, and royalty wore crystal-laden crowns to stimulate enlightenment and awaken their third eyes. The most coveted stones in ancient Egypt were Carnelian, Clear Quartz, Emerald, Lapis Lazuli, Peridot, and Turquoise.

CHINA

In ancient China, healing crystals were commonly used in Chinese medicine, including crystal-tipped needles in acupuncture healing sessions, fêng shui, adornment, home décor, musical instruments, and armor and weapons. Some of these crystal traditions in China go back as far as eight thousand years, and many are still in use today. Jade was and still is the fave!

GREECE

The word *crystal* is derived from the Greek word *krystallos,* which means "clear ice." Legend has it that ancient Greeks believed Clear Quartz crystals were ice sent from the heavens. Ancient Greek warriors rubbed crushed Hematite on their bodies as a pre-battle ritual to make themselves invincible. The myth of how Amethyst got its name is a story about Dionysus, Greek god of wine and the grape harvest, and his obsession with a girl named Amethystos. Amethystos wasn't interested in Dionysus and opted to "swipe left," praying to the goddess Artemis to keep Dionysus away from her at all costs. Artemis's solution was to transform Amethystos into a white stone as permanent protection. It is said that Dionysus then poured wine over the stone as an offering, dyeing the crystal purple (an alternate legend has it that he was so upset about losing Amethystos, he cried tears of wine, staining the stone purple). The word *amethyst* comes from the Greek *amethystos*, meaning "without drunkenness," and in modern-day crystal medicine, it is used to help people with addiction issues.

INDIA

Ayurveda, the traditional Hindu system of medicine, considers crystals invaluable for healing emotional and metaphysical imbalances and to counteract the effects of our personal astrology and karma. We can find reference to this within the pages of one of the oldest Hindu scripts, the Vedas, which reference each stone's specific healing abilities.

JAPAN

In ancient Japan, Clear Quartz crystal balls were used by Buddhist monks in the art of scrying. These practitioners believed Crystal Quartz held the powers of the "dragon heart," allowing its user to harness the power and wisdom of the dragon for increased "second sight" through prophecy and spirit communication.

NEW ZEALAND

The Maoris of New Zealand have long worn Jade pendants to honor ancestor spirits, and they still consider Jade to be a stone of luck today.

THE AMAZONS

The legendary Amazon women of Greek mythology were supposedly man-hating matriarchs. The women would visit nearby tribes once a year to procreate, and they sent all baby boys away to be cared for elsewhere. To prepare for battle later in life, the right breasts of all Amazon infants were seared off to improve their archery skills. That's hard core! However, these fearless female warriors still took the time to enjoy the beauty and benefits of crystals. Archaeologists believe the Amazons descended from the Scythian people, and they discovered the ancient burial mound of a Scythian woman they dubbed the "Siberian Ice Princess." Covered in tattoos and wearing a silk shirt and jewelry, she appeared to be a decorated warrior, a well-dressed princess, and a holy woman to boot. Buried with her were a wig, a cosmetic compact, and—you guessed it—makeup pigments made of ground crystals. The blue-green stone Amazonite, known as the "Stone of Courage and Truth," is named for these ancient lady-warriors. Legend says that these warrior babes would rub their wounds with crushed Amazonite to avoid infection, and they would decorate their armor with the stone and carry it with them at all times for increased protection.

NATIVE AMERICANS

The indigenous people of the Americas considered crystals to be important teaching tools and used them for healing, and in burial rites, ceremonies, celebrations, and life-marking events. They also believed that each gemstone represented a different Spirit Animal.

WHY CRYSTALS ARE SO POWERFUL

People have been attracted to crystals since the dawn of time for burial rites, divination practices, healing rituals, spiritual advancement, and as decoration to connote power. Our ancestors intuitively knew that crystals could bring about energetic shifts and changes, whether worn as adornment, kept in close proximity, or used in ritual. People have also long gravitated toward sites like Stonehenge and Sedona because these massive rock formations are powerful energy vortexes.

Let's put some facts behind the "ancient woo" by discussing how science and mysticism intersect. We know that crystals are millions of years old, forged during the earliest part of the earth's formation. I be-

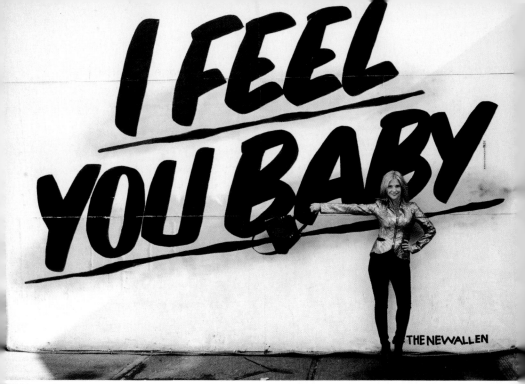

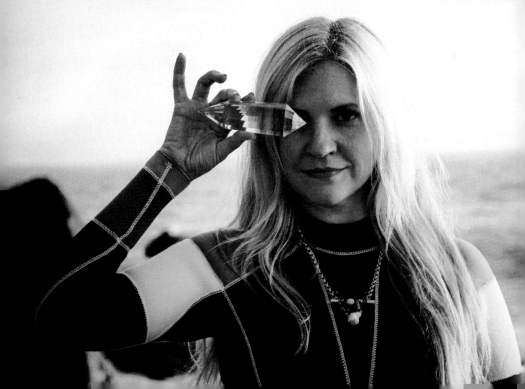

lieve that crystals are a timeless database of knowledge, because they retain all the information they have ever been exposed to. Crystals absorb information, whether a severe weather pattern or the experience of an ancient ceremony, and pass this information along to the next person who comes into contact with them.

Scientifically, crystals are the most orderly structure that exists in nature. Crystals are structured in such a way that they respond to the different energies that surround them by oscillating and emitting specific vibratory frequencies. The way they are balanced, the frequencies they emit, and their ability to store a tremendous amount of information makes crystals essential to modern technology. This is why crystals are used in computers, TVs, cell phones, satellites, electricity, and just about every tech-y item that exists in the modern world.

GOING VOGEL

The crystal shape I find to be the most powerful is the Vogel-Cut, a multifaceted Clear Quartz crystal named for its creator, Marcel Vogel (1917–1991). The Vogel crystal is considered by crystal practitioners to be an instrument that can amplify, convert, and store subtle energies. Vogel was a research scientist at IBM for twenty-eight years, and his areas of expertise were liquid crystal systems, luminescence, phosphor technology, and magnetics. He retired from IBM in 1984 and founded his own laboratory, Psychic Research, Inc., where he delved into crystal research and more esoteric fields of study, and spent the last years of his career studying the relationship between quartz crystals and water. His theories on crystals have often been dismissed as "metaphysical" by the scientific community, but it is interesting to note that IBM donated more than $500,000 in equipment to fund Vogel's independent crystal research after he left the company. Vogel's greatest goal in his work was to prove that the scientific and metaphysical were not only compatible, but could work and play together for the greater good of humanity.

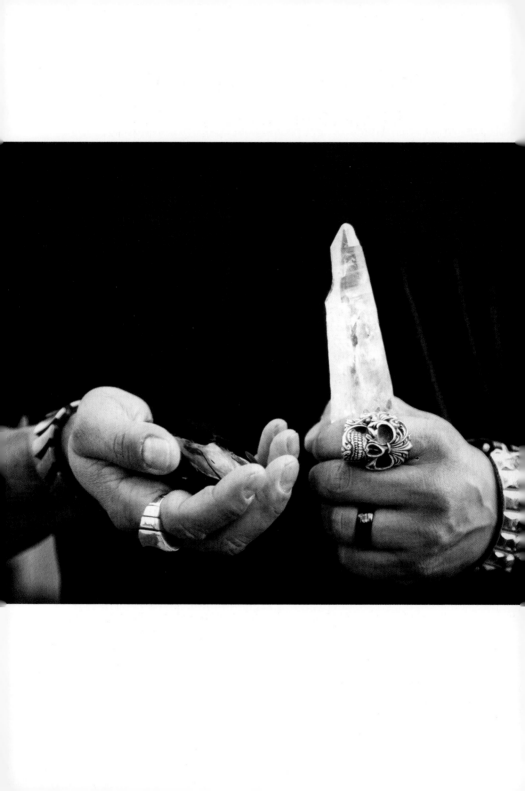

Interview with a Silicon Valley Engineer on Crystals and Technology

I WAS FORTUNATE ENOUGH to meet with a Silicon Valley engineer at a leading technology company whose job is soooo top secret that we had to maintain his anonymity. He's an inventor who has helped bring us some really cool products. This technologist is not only one of the loveliest, coolest, and most talented people I have ever met but also happens to be one of the smartest. Besides his pedigree with his company, his accolades include being one of the key inventors of the GPS technology used in cell phones, being one of the smartest physicists in the world, and designing guitars in his free time. Mind officially blown! I must admit, I was a little nervous about our convo. How were a man of science and a girl from the mystical fringe going to "communicate" about crystals? The first thing he said to me when we met was, "If it weren't for crystals, we would still be living in the 1950s." I relaxed and knew we were about to have an epic conversation. Do you recognize these hands?

What do you do professionally?

In a nutshell, I get to play with some of the most brilliant people on the planet, and as a result, we help create products that we're crazy passionate about.

When we met, you said something quite impactful to me: "If it weren't for crystals, we would still be living in the 1950s." Can you explain why crystals are important in technology?

Colleen, how can I put this? Crystals are not important in technology. They *are* technology. Without our use of crystals and crystal structures, which constitute every single microchip ever made, humanity as we know it today would not exist in the same way. My precious cell phone and computer would not exist. Our flat-screen TVs and computerized cars and autopilot planes and intelligent software that it takes to create our modern roads and complex distribution systems would not exist. Our state-of-the-art buildings and cutting-edge architectural structures and mind-blowing advancements in medicine and the sequencing of the human genome and everything in between: We would not have these things today without our use of miniaturized high-speed computing systems, and at the heart of every computer there is at least one microchip. And guess what. A microchip is a sliver of a man-made crystal with elaborate structures built on it. So to put it bluntly, crystals are a fundamental building block to our civilization as we know it today.

The advent of the microchip is much more profound than most people realize. Up until the 1950s, we built computers out of vacuum tubes, punch cards, and levers, which meant computers were physically large. It wasn't until humanity created solid-state transistors that we were able to shrink the vacuum tube from the size of a Popsicle (without the stick) to the size of a Tic Tac. But even that wasn't enough to be able to get us to where we are now. It wasn't until the 1960s that pioneers at Texas Instruments and Fairchild really paved the way to building transistors on germanium and silicon crystal structures, respectively.

Today, Wikipedia states that a cell phone's microprocessor contains 4.3 billion transistors in it, on crystal substrates that are essentially about 88 square millimeters. That is smaller than the area of your thumbnail. If we were to try to create the same computer out of 4.3 billion Popsicle-size vacuum tubes that are 1.5 inches in diameter by 4 inches tall, it would require a space of about 16.8 million cubic feet. That's a room measuring 256 feet wide by 256 feet long by 256 feet tall. Nobody would be able to store this thing.

Today, I pay between $30 and $80 for a vacuum tube for one of my guitar amps. Even if I could get a vacuum tube for a penny, this vacuum-tube-based system would cost me $4.3 million. But that's just the main processor. These calculations don't take into account all of the other supporting circuitry—microchips and components and assemblies and whatnot. Without crystals, almost every computer that we use today would be unaffordable, unable to be mass-produced, rendering them unobtainable and incapable of being stored by the average person. And did I forget to mention how much power it would require to operate such a beast? You'd probably have to sell your home for a month of use.

So when I hear people say that their computer-based product is expensive or too big or doesn't hold as much of a charge as they'd like it to, they just don't have perspective on where we came from and where we are now. It's because of the use of crystals that modern-day technology is what it is today.

Where else do we find crystals? Energy drinks, electric guitars, etc. Places people wouldn't normally think of . . . like, aside from an altar ;)

I've come to realize that the word *crystal* refers more to the ordered structure of an object or system rather than the object itself. Metals can be crystallized. Elements in a gaseous state can be formed into crystals. Even certain ceramic materials can have their molecules arranged in such an orderly fashion that they exhibit some piezoelectric properties just like real crystals.

One might even go so far as to say that a crystal is the thing that nature has revealed to us as being as close to our concept of perfection as we can currently observe. It is because of this extreme intimacy with perfection that mankind creates crystals today. Due to the highly ordered structure of a crystal, we are capable of precisely predicting the events, movements, and locations of the molecules that constitute that crystal. This allows us the ability to mathematically model and alter these ordered objects with a very high degree of accuracy. As a result, we are able to design and manufacture technological devices that make use of crystals with high degrees of reproducibility, repeatability, and reliability; companies worldwide do it in the billions. Crystals in technology have indeed already helped almost every living human on the face of this earth in one way or another; it's just not that evident to people that that's what's been going on.

If you were a crystal, which crystal would you be?

I'd have to be a sugar crystal.

CRYSTAL BATHING: SCIENCE WRAPPED UP IN A MYSTICAL BOW

How do modern day healers work with Vogel crystals? They primarily use these crystals for healing, meditation, channeling, and to remove mental, physical, emotional, and energetic toxins from the body. These toxins may be described by healers and clients alike as dense, tense, sticky, negative, dark, nagging, or heavy feelings. A Vogel crystal is cut with the intention to amplify, coalesce, and focus any energies you wish to direct into someone's body or mind. The design of the crystal allows for your thoughts and energy to enter the crystal at the receptive end, be amplified and focused as it travels in a circular pattern through the crystal, and be transmitted like a laser beam from the focal end.

The most remarkable example of how Vogel crystals are used is in crystal beds, also known as John of God beds or crystal bath therapy. These beds were originally created by world-renowned healer John of God, and used by his team of spirit doctors at the Casa de Dom Inácio in Brazil. The beds have also been adopted by other healers around the world and are used for alignment, rejuvenation, and balancing of energy fields, which in turn aids energetic and physical healing.

What is a treatment with one of these beds like? The client lies on a massage table, and a metal arm with seven clear, highly polished Vogel quartz crystals suspended from it swings over the client's body. Each crystal is cut to a specific frequency and is energetically aligned above one of the seven main chakras. Colored lights, which match the vibrational frequency of the chakra colors—red, orange, yellow, green, blue, indigo, and purple—radiate through each crystal onto the client's body in blinking rhythms to cleanse, balance, and align energy. The individual receiving the session lies faceup, with eyes closed, bathing in the energy for 10 to 60 minutes. I have had crystal bed treatments many times and can best describe what I have felt as tingles and vibrations throughout my body.

CRYSTALS ON THE BRAIN AND IN THE BODY

Crystals are not only vital to operate our iPhones. Incredibly, they may also be essential for our bodies to function. Dr. Joseph Kirschvink, a professor at the California Institute of Technology, claims we actually have crystals in our brains! According to Dr. Kirschvink, human brain cells possess a highly magnetic mineral known as Magnetite, which acts like a tiny internal compass to help us find our way. Magnetite can also be found in animals that use magnetoreception to guide them: homing pigeons, migratory salmon, dolphins, honeybees, dogs, moths, and bats. Scientists at the California Institute of Technology discovered that humans have a tiny piece of Magnetite in the ethmoid bone, which is located between our eyes, just behind the nose. Magnetite is the most magnetic substance on the planet, and this piece is coincidentally located within the nose at the exact location where mystics believe our telepathic senses sit. Science has even acknowledged that Magnetite could be linked to telepathy. This also happens to be the same region where the pineal gland, aka the Third-Eye Chakra, is located.

We also keep our balance thanks to calcium carbonate crystals, aka "ear rocks," embedded in our inner ear. If these tiny inner crystals become dislodged, it can lead to vertigo. Additionally, we are able to stand up straight because of calcium phosphate crystals that reinforce our skeletons. And we have crystals to thank for our smiles—our pearly whites are made of apatite microcrystals. Not to mention that piezo crystals are found in your teeth, bones, intestines, tendons, ligaments, and cartilage as well as in record needles and electric guitars.

WE ARE ALL BECOMING X-MEN BECAUSE OF CRYSTALS!

Both scientists and mystics alike believe we are moving from carbon-based beings to crystalline-based beings because our "junk DNA" is activating. Puzzled? Let me explain?

Science

Geneticists believe we are going through an evolutionary leap. The human body has the potential to carry four to twelve strands of DNA. The more strands of DNA we carry, the more intelligent or intuitive we become. A convention of geneticists from around the world stated that soon, we will be developing twelve-strand DNA helixes. Each extra strand of DNA will grant us "superhuman" abilities that might be considered paranormal. Scientists suggest that there is more to DNA than just storing our genetic info—that by activating our DNA beyond the current two strands, we become connected to higher frequencies and activate dormant abilities, such as clairvoyance, telepathy, and multidimensional consciousness.

Mystics

Spiritualists believe that the activation of our higher strands of DNA will allow our bodies to process more data and expand our consciousness. A healthy human brain processes 400 billion plus bits of information per second. Currently we are only using two thousand of those 400 billion bits daily. Our conscious mind currently allows us to be aware of 1 percent of reality, leaving the rest of the information to be processed by our subconscious mind. As we evolve, we will continue to activate all the functionalities associated with our sixth sense in a more present manner.

If both camps are correct, we may be quickly evolving and activating the higher DNA strands that could be the key to enlightenment. So what does it mean to have a "crystalline body"? A great example is when a log burns down and all that remains is the element carbon. If a diamond is placed in a fire, its structure is retained. Our cells must be transformed from carbon to a silicon crystal so that we can withstand the tremendous amount of "light," as spiritualists would say, or energy, as scientists would say, that our bodies can hold. Internally, all our cells are being changed from an organic structure to a crystalline structure, which is the perfect prism through which light can pass. As we evolve, we will be able to hold and process more light in our bodies, becoming higher-frequency beings.

Are scientists and mystics both picking up on the same hot spots in the body, but communicating about the subject in different ways? Are crystals not only helping us with practical, linear functions like balance and eating, but also acting as a built-in generator for telepathy and following our inner compass?

Now that you know the who, what, where, when, and how of your most precious, magical gems, let's RSVP *YES!* to curating an entire runway-worthy collection in the next chapter.

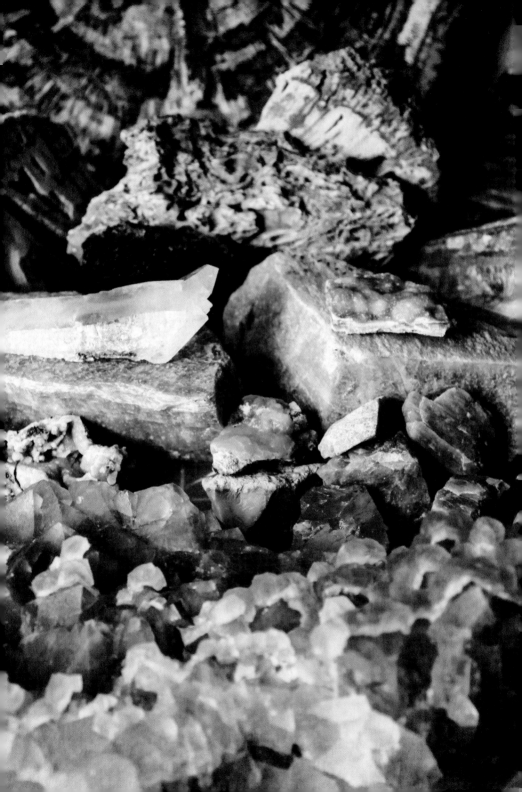

4

YOUR MINI ENCYCLOPEDIA OF CRYSTALS

Buy what you don't have yet, or what you really want, which can be mixed with what you already own. Buy only because something excites you, not just for the simple act of shopping.

–KARL LAGERFELD

CONGRATULATIONS! You've graduated from beginner status, and now you're ready to go from dabbler to collector. You of course don't need to go out and buy everything on this list all at once! But use it as a point of reference as you build on your crystal basics (kind of like you would build on the basics in your wardrobe!), and make it your go-to when you want to take your crystal kit to the next level. This list mirrors my own collection, which I've carefully curated over the years based on wisdom I've gained from my mentors and my personal work with stones. Like the Top 20 Stones (see pages 59–77), each of these graduate-level stones comes with an extensive list of mental, physical, spiritual, and emotional benefits, but I've chosen to address just the highlights here, along with the most interesting mystical lore and the ways I use them in my private sessions with clients.

1. Agate

AKA: "The Character Builder"

The Look: Every color of the Pantone rainbow

Where It Comes From: Argentina, Australia, Botswana, Brazil, India, Poland, Mexico, Uruguay, United States

The "C Spot": All

Why You Need It in Your Life: In ancient times, Agate was used to ward off storms. Today, we work with Agate to call on extra physical strength and emotional endurance when navigating the sh*tstorms of life.

Mystical Homework: It's been one of those days. Hold Agate in your hand while you binge-watch Netflix and eat ice cream.

Crystal Affirmation:: "I will weather the storm."

2. Amazonite

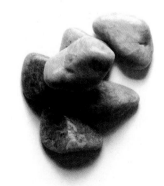

AKA: "The Task Master"

The Look: Blue-green

Where It Comes From: Brazil, India, Ethiopia, Myanmar, Madagascar, Russia, United States

The "C Spot": 4th/Heart Chakra and 5th/Throat Chakra

Why You Need It in Your Life: Amazonite is associated with the astrological sign Virgo. This stone helps with organization, thinking practically, and making grounded decisions, in true Virgo fashion.

Mystical Homework: Hold this stone while making your to-do list.

Crystal Affirmation: "I am organized."

3. Apache Tears

AKA: "Cry It Out"

The Look: Shiny black

Where It Comes From: United States

The "C Spot": 1st/Root Chakra

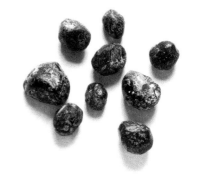

Why You Need It in Your Life: Apache Tears help to clear negative thoughts that you may be having about yourself or others, or that others are sending in your direction. This stone combats gossip, lies, jealousy, greed, resentment, and bullying. Accept that these negative thought-forms exist and then release them.

Mystical Homework: Get the dense energy out of your body by getting physical. Take your Apache Tears to a boxing class and imagine that you-know-who's face is on the heavy bag. With every punch, take a deep breath and release emotionally sticky energy and thoughts, and your mind will be clearer after the class, allowing you to better handle your emotions when you're not in the ring.

Crystal Affirmation: "I will allow negative thoughts and actions to float away."

4. Aqua Aura Quartz

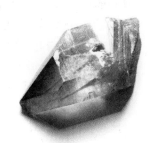

AKA: "The High-Vibe Heavyweight"

The Look: Blue as a cloudless day in LA

Where It Comes From: Brazil, Canada, China, Germany, Madagascar, Peru, South Africa, United States

The "C Spot": All, but particularly the 6th/Third-Eye Chakra and 7th/Crown Chakra

Why You Need It in Your Life: Aqua Aura Quartz enhances mental clarity and allows you to connect with the unseen with confidence. It activates and enhances psychic awareness, clairaudience, clairvoyance, clairsentience, claircognizance, and "automatic writing" skills (writing that is said to be produced by a spiritual or subconscious agency acting through you, as opposed to by your conscious intention). It also helps you communicate with your Spirit Guides, and it activates all your chakras so they can work together like a well-oiled machine.

Mystical Homework: Place Aqua Aura Quartz on your third eye to connect with your inherent sixth sense. We all have sixth-sense perception, to some degree, which basically means the ability to perceive the world beyond the basic five senses (hearing, sight, smell, taste, and touch).

Crystal Affirmation: "I connect with confidence."

5. Aquamarine

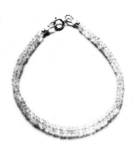

AKA: "Seaworthy"

The Look: Tiffany blue

Where It Comes From: Angola, Brazil, Kenya,

Madagascar, Malawi, Mozambique, Nigeria, Pakistan, Russia, Tanzania, United States, Zambia

The "C Spot": 5th/Throat Chakra

Why You Need It in Your Life: Aquamarine was believed to be the treasure of mermaids and was used as a sailor's good-luck talisman, according to mystical lore. It opens the watery channels of emotion for self-reflection and better communication with others.

Mystical Homework: Wear a bracelet made of Aquamarine while boating or sailing the high seas to boost the qualities mentioned above.

Crystal Affirmation: "I am a reflection for what the universe mirrors back to me."

6. Astrophyllite

AKA: "The Divine Blueprint"

The Look: Shiny with variations of brown, golden yellow, and green

Where It Comes From: Canada, Greenland, Norway, Russia, United States

The "C Spot": All

Why You Need It in Your Life: This stone carries a direct and potent message best embodied by the ancient Greek aphorism "Know thyself," which was inscribed on the Oracle of Delphi's temple. Astrophyllite facilitates self-knowledge, self-realization, self-acceptance, reclaiming personal power, and facing one's deepest fears (known in Jungian philosophy as "the shadow") head on. Working with Astrophyllite isn't about coming up with your five-year plan. It's about confronting the bigger picture of your life in a cosmic sense, and finding your soul's purpose.

Mystical Homework: Do not touch this stone unless you are ready to step up and make some big life changes. I bought one of these and shortly thereafter moved across the country and changed careers. True story.

Crystal Affirmation: "I am ready."

7. Black Kyanite

AKA: "The Witch's Broom"

The Look: Black-hole black

Where It Comes From: Austria, Brazil, Italy, Kenya, Switzerland

The "C Spot": All

Why You Need It in Your Life: Black Kyanite sweeps energetic dust out of all the chakras and can repair holes and tears in the auric field. It is a superior grounding stone as it activates the Earth-Star Chakra (which is about one foot below your feet).

Mystical Homework: While in a standing position, place Black Kyanite on the floor between your feet to provide extra grounding of your spiritual energy. Take some really deep yoga-style breaths and visualize your feet having tiny little roots that are sinking into the earth.

Crystal Affirmation: "Any energy that does not serve my highest and greatest good, get the f*** out (with love)."

8. Blue Apatite

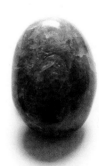

AKA: "Balance the Scales"

The Look: Blue

Where It Comes From: Brazil, Canada, India,

Kenya, Madagascar, Mexico, Myanmar, Norway, South Africa, Sri Lanka, United States

The "C Spot": 5th/Throat Chakra

Why You Need It in Your Life: You won't forget this one: Apatite is an appetite suppressant! It regulates problematic eating issues, encourages healthy eating habits, raises your metabolic rate, works as an immune system booster, and heals the glands and organs.

Mystical Homework: Hold on to this stone for dear life while dieting, juicing, or on a cleanse. You've got this!

Crystal Affirmation: "I do not want that double chocolate chip filled-with-gluten-and-goodness cookie!"

9. Blue Kyanite

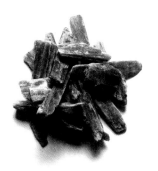

AKA: "The Psychic Hotline"

The Look: Sapphire-like blue streaked with white

Where It Comes From: Brazil, Kenya, Russia, Switzerland, Tanzania, United States

The "C Spot": 6th/Third-Eye Chakra and 7th/Crown Chakra

Why You Need It in Your Life: Blue Kyanite is a self-cleansing stone that can activate psychic gifts, provide an energetic armor around the body, and instantly align the chakras. This is a great stone for healers and those just getting into the esoteric arts.

Mystical Homework: Meditate while lying down, and place a piece of Blue Kyanite over your third eye, as this is where we connect with our psychic intuition within our bodies. This practice helps to awaken your third eye.

Crystal Affirmation: "I trust my intuition."

10. Celestite

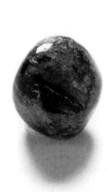

AKA: "The Big Guns"

The Look: Sparkly sky blue

Where It Comes From: Madagascar, United States

The "C Spot": 6th/Third-Eye Chakra

Why You Need It in Your Life:
Looking for a little extra guidance? This stone helps you connect to and communicate with your Spirit Guides, whoever they may be. Everyone's guides are different. Whether you prefer to seek guidance from God in the traditional monotheistic sense, from various gods and goddesses, from angels, priestesses, spirit animals, universal energy, or your grandmother who has crossed over, this stone will help.

Mystical Homework: Wishing you could just text your Spirit Guides in a pinch? Try sitting quietly in your sacred space while holding Celestite and asking them to show themselves. Then wait for them to start communicating.

Crystal Affirmation: "I am asking for guidance."

11. Charoite

AKA: "The Force"

The Look: Purple with hints of white, black, lilac, and brown

Where It Comes From: Russia

The "C Spot": 4th/Heart Chakra and 7th/Crown Chakra

Why You Need It in Your Life: Ideal if you're a practitioner just getting into the crystal healing game. Charoite assists healers in being of service and being objective about the information they receive from a client, in order to ensure that they are reading the client's energy and issues, not their own. It also prevents psychic burnout.

Mystical Homework: Having trouble getting a read on how a meeting with a client, your boss, or your colleagues went? Trust in Charoite—it's in the "client services" business. Hold this stone while meditating and ask your Spirit Guides to help you home in on what went wrong or right and what the best next steps are to take in the boardroom.

Crystal Affirmation: "I practice discernment with clear and healthy boundaries."

12. Chrysanthemum Stone

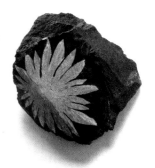

AKA: "Lady Luck"

The Look: Chalkboard black with a white flower pattern

Where It Comes From: Canada, China, Japan, United States

The "C Spot": All

Why You Need It in Your Life: This stone encourages luck, synchronicity, and achieving your fullest potential. It is known to increase both the number and frequency of fortuitous "coincidences" in your life. In other words, it helps you to get in the flow so divine timing can work on your behalf.

Mystical Homework: Carry it in your pocket and use it as a worry stone if you feel like the sun is always shining on the opposite side of the street.

Crystal Affirmation: "I walk in blind faith."

13. Copper

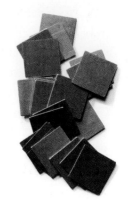

AKA: "Pump Up the Volume"

The Look: Copper

Where It Comes From: Chile, Indonesia, Peru, United States

The "C Spot": All

Why You Need It in Your Life:
Discovered in 9000 BC, Copper, like all metals, is a great conductor of energy. Though it's not a stone or a crystal, I'm including Copper on this list because of its ability to conduct and amplify energy between people, between different crystals, and between the mind and the spirit world. Copper is an amazing accoutrement or accessory to set next to any crystal you want to amplify the vibration of. It's also believed to help regrow joint cartilage.

Mystical Homework: Wear a Copper bracelet to not only reduce joint pain, but amplify the vibes of all your crystal bangles.

Crystal Affirmation: "I want to amplify _____ through my thoughts, words, and actions." (Fill in the blank: positivity, love, emotional support, etc.)

14. Dalmatian Stone

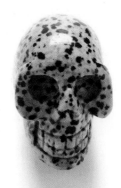

AKA: "The Anti–Hamster Wheel"

The Look: Literally looks like a Dalmatian

Where It Comes From: Australia, Brazil, India, Indonesia, Egypt, Kazakhstan, Madagascar, Uruguay, Venezuela, United States

The "C Spot": 1st/Root Chakra

Why You Need It in Your Life: Does any of the following sound familiar? You can't silence obsessive or looping thoughts in your mind. You can't stop thinking about your ever-growing to-do list, your overflowing inbox, and all the people you have to call. You constantly worry over whether you've made a good first impression. You check your phone like Pavlov's dog every time it pings. If you answered yes to any of these, this is the stone for you!

Mystical Homework: Create your own personal Sabbath with this "Supreme Nurturer" stone. Take a day off (Saturday and Sunday are usually best for this), rest, and celebrate! Turn off your phone, light a few candles, invite your nearest and dearest over, and just connect.

Crystal Affirmation: "I don't need to look at my phone!"

15. Danburite

AKA: "Crystal Drano"

The Look: Clear and colorless

Where It Comes From: Bolivia, Japan, Madagascar, Myanmar, Russia, United States

The "C Spot": 4th/Crown, 6th/Third-Eye, and 7th/Heart Chakra

Why You Need It in Your Life: Danburite alleviates blockages on all levels (except maybe traffic on the 405). Relieves allergies, digestive issues, and muscle tension, as well as emotional congestion, karmic wounds, self-pride, and negative thinking.

Mystical Homework: Feeling stress in your shoulders? Lay down and place Danburite on your sore muscles to start to break up the knots.

Crystal Affirmation: "I release my issues."

16. Druzy

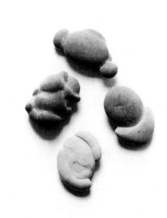

AKA: "The Social Butterfly"

The Look: All colors, depending on what the crystal cluster is bonded to

Where It Comes From: Druzy can form in any location where there is a place for water to collect and evaporate on rock.

The "C Spot":: All, again depending on the stone it bonds to

Why You Need It in Your Life: A Druzy (also known as Druse or Drusy) is a coating of fine crystals on a fractured rock surface. Since Druzies grow in clusters, they are social stones that are ideal for use during group gatherings like work meetings, parties, or Moon Circles.

Mystical Homework: Wear Druzy jewelry whenever you are out and about so you can attract your like-minded tribe.

Crystal Affirmation: "I am a social butterfly."

17. Fairy Stone

AKA: "Mother Earth Protector"

The Look: Gray

Where It Comes From: Canada

The "C Spot": 1st/Root Chakra and 7th/Crown Chakra

Why You Need It in Your Life: Native Americans traditionally kept Fairy Stone in the home to promote health, prosperity, luck on hunts, protection from evil spirits, and to appease the spirits. This stone encourages us to give thanks and to care for the well-being of our Earth.

Mystical Homework: Love Mama Earth and remember to recycle!

Crystal Affirmation: "Thank you for holding me, Pachamama." (Pachamama is a fertility goddess of the indigenous people of the Andes who embodies "Mother Earth.")

18. Fire Lemurian Quartz

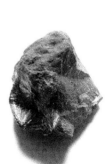

AKA: "The Fire Starter"

The Look: Smoky to clear with a dusting of red or pink tones

Where It Comes From: Brazil

The "C Spot": All

Why You Need It in Your Life: According to metaphysical lore, these stones contain ancient wisdom from the lost civilization of Lemuria (somewhat similar to Atlantis). Holding this stone is said to ignite this ancient wisdom. These "master crystals" are associated with all the chakras, all astrological signs, all elements, and all the planets.

Mystical Homework: Think of this crystal as a portable library of all that ever was. If you want to get in on ancient wisdom (like Yoda, Gandalf, and Mr. Miyagi), try meditating with this crystal in your left hand.

Crystal Affirmation: "I ask for access to ancient wisdom."

19. Galena

AKA: "The Harmonizer"

The Look: Shiny, metallic silver

Where It Comes From: Austria, Belgium, France, Italy, Romania, United States

The "C Spot": 1st/Root Chakra

Why You Need It in Your Life: Galena is a stone of harmony that helps banish self-limiting beliefs and negative self-talk by absorbing the personal negativity you are holding on to.

Mystical Homework: Galena contains materials that cannot be kept next to skin, so it is best used on a shelf or sacred space, instead of as a hand-held meditation stone. On a full moon, make a list of all the things that are holding you back from being the best version of yourself. Stick Galena on top of the list until the next full moon. Then have your own personal "releasing ceremony" by burning the list. Say adieu to what is no longer serving you. P.S. Always wash your hands after handing this stone.

Crystal Affirmation: "I am anything I want to be."

20. Girasol

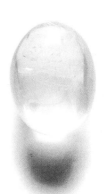

AKA: "The Myth Buster"

The Look: Opalescent with a soap-opera-lighting glow

Where It Comes From: Madagascar

The "C Spot": 6th/Third-Eye Chakra

Why You Need It in Your Life: Midway between Quartz and Opal, Girasol is an ancient stone of transformation, and it should be used in times of life transition. It helps us to see through illusions, to see ourselves and others more clearly, and to recognize what is being "mirrored" back at us by others.

Mystical Homework: Meditate with this stone and ask your Spirit Guides to show you some truth in yourself that you are unaware of. A cold, hard look in the mirror can be tough, but it's totally worth it.

Crystal Affirmation: "I see through my own bullsh*t and the bullsh*t of others."

21. Green Aventurine

AKA: "The Money Maker"

The Look: Green like a lucky shamrock

Where It Comes From: Austria, Brazil, Chile, India, Spain, Tanzania, Russia

The "C Spot": 4th/Heart Chakra

Why You Need It in Your Life: Want to call in more money, honey? This is the "Stone of Opportunity," prosperity, wealth, winning competitions and bets, and basically coming out on top.

Mystical Homework: Get crafty and build a "Financial Abundance" crystal grid using Aventurine, Jade, Citrine, Green Moss Agate, Iron Pyrite, and Clear Quartz (see the section on Crystal Gridding in chapter 5 for more detail on how to do this). Extra credit if you put it in the Wealth section of your home according to fêng shui principles. The number 8 in numerology represents financial power, so work that into the grid, too. Arrange your grid on the new moon, as this is a day when we call in what we want in our lives.

Crystal Affirmation: "I will accumulate abundance."

22. Hematite

AKA: "The Trip Advisor"

The Look: Metallic gray

Where It Comes From: Australia, Brazil, China, India, South Africa, Russia, Ukraine, United States

The "C Spot": 1st/Root Chakra

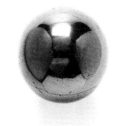

Why You Need It in Your Life: Hematite protects and strengthens the body during stressful moments, like when you're encountering turbulence on a flight, for example. It's known for being the stone in the crystal kingdom with the most "gravity," which makes it good for grounding. It's an especially useful stone for relieving stress during travel, and it is *the* stone for combating jet lag.

Mystical Homework: Keep it in your carry-on.

Crystal Affirmation: "I am grounded."

23. Herkimer Diamond

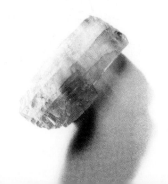

AKA: "A Girl's Best Friend"

The Look: Clear and colorless

Where It Comes From: Canada, China, England, Germany, United States (The Mohawk Indians and early settlers of Herkimer, New York, and the surrounding area were the first to discover this crystal, hence its name.)

The "C Spot": 6th (and up)/Third-Eye Chakra

Why You Need It in Your Life: Herkimer Diamond is like a booster shot of inner sparkle. This stone will leave you feeling radiant, energized, light, limitless, and youthful, and it can increase your dream recall.

Mystical Homework: Feeling adventurous? Take a field trip to the crystal mines in Herkimer, New York, and dig one up yourself.

Crystal Affirmation: "I shine bright like a Herkimer Diamond."

24. Hiddenite

AKA: "Cupid's Arrow"

The Look: Glassy pale green, yellow-green, or emerald green

Where It Comes From: Afghanistan, Brazil, China, Madagascar, Myanmar, Pakistan, United States

The "C Spot": 4th/Heart Chakra

Why You Need It in Your Life: This one is all about love, baby! Hiddenite awakens your heart, helping you to attract true love, proclaim love for someone else, reignite love that feels stagnant, and dissolve emotional blockages in the heart.

Mystical Homework: Place Hiddenite on your heart center. In your mind's eye, picture all your nearest and dearest, and send out some love to them.

Crystal Affirmation: "I am a mirror for the love I want to attract."

25. Howlite

AKA: "Whoa, Nelly!"

The Look: Snow white with gray speckles

Where It Comes From: Canada

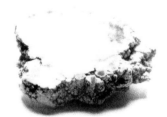

The "C Spot": All

Why You Need It in Your Life: But how? This stone is for you if you constantly find yourself in overdrive, your mind going a thousand miles a minute, thinking, *How is this going to get done or fixed or made or delivered?* If you're looking to slow your overactive mind, Howlite is for you! It also relieves muscle tension (you overworked stressball). It's an "attunement" stone, meaning it opens the mind to receiving information and wisdom.

Mystical Homework: Challenge yourself to embrace a week-long technology detox.

Crystal Affirmation: "It's okay to slow down!"

26. Iceland Spar (Optical Calcite)

AKA: "Double Vision"

The Look: Clear and colorless

Where It Comes From: Iceland

The "C Spot": All

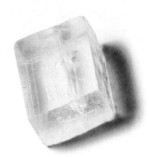

Why You Need It in Your Life: The Vikings called this "sunstone" and used it as a navigation tool for finding the sun in overcast weather conditions because of its polarizing effect. Iceland Spar (Optical Calcite) is a double-refractive stone, meaning that items viewed through it will appear as if they are in two places at once, creating a double image. This "Stone of the Mind" broadens our perceptions and opens us up to seeing hidden meanings behind actions and words. It also helps heal eye conditions.

Mystical Homework: Lay this stone over the top of printed words and watch the magic of seeing double.

Crystal Affirmation: "I am open to seeing both sides of a situation."

27. Iolite

AKA: "The Phoenix"

The Look: Purple or blue

Where It Comes From: Brazil, Canada, India, Madagascar, Myanmar, Namibia, Sri Lanka, Tanzania, United States

The "C Spot": 6th/Third-Eye Chakra

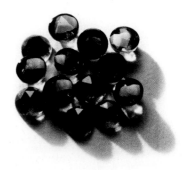

Why You Need It in Your Life: You've just been through a rough patch, but like a phoenix, you are ready to rise from the ashes and get yourself back on track. Also known as the "Stone of the Muses," Iolite will inspire you to restore life balance, harness your personal power, settle debts, and work through addictions.

Mystical Homework: To help curb addictions and cravings, carry a tumbled Iolite "worry stone" in your pocket or handbag. It's like having a tiny supportive cheerleader close by. Iolite works especially well for combating addictions like drugs, alcohol, financial debt, overspending, and gambling.

Crystal Affirmation: "I will rise again."

28. Larvikite

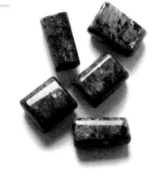

AKA: "The Stone of Grounded Magic"
The Look: Marbled black and gray
Where It Comes From: Canada, India, Norway
The "C Spot": 1st/Root Chakra
Why You Need It in Your Life: Also known as the "Norwegian Pearl," as it originated from the Larvik region of Norway, Larvikite helps to establish an unbreakable "wisdom exchange" between the user and the spiritual realm. It also opens up new pathways of knowledge in the brain, assists us with taking in new info more easily, and makes us feel more secure about the strength of our intellect.

Mystical Homework: Want to figure out who your Spirit Guides are? While meditating with Larvikite in your hand, ask the universe, "Universe, who is personally guiding me on my path from the unseen realms?" In response, you may hear a name, see a face, or just get a feeling of a presence in your personal space.

Crystal Affirmation: "I am a seeker of everyday, practical, grounded magic."

29. Pink Mangano Calcite

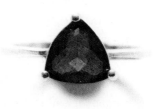

AKA: "Hot Hands"

The Look: Pink and white

Where It Comes From: Belgium, Brazil, Bulgaria, Mexico, Peru

The "C Spot": 4th/Heart Chakra

Why You Need It in Your Life: This is the official stone of Reiki (a technique where the practitioner uses their hands to promote healing). This stone promotes qualities that we typically associate with Reiki treatments: peace, well-being, gentleness, calm, and unconditional love for yourself and others. Pink Mangano Calcite is also a heart opener, aids in sleep, and releases tension and suppressed emotion.

Mystical Homework: Book yourself a Reiki session and ask your practitioner about Pink Mangano Calcite.

Crystal Affirmation: "I am calm."

30. Moldavite

AKA: "The Cosmonaut"

The Look: Forest or olive green

Where It Comes From: Czech Republic

The "C Spot": 4th/Heart Chakra

Why You Need It in Your Life: Moldavite formed as the result of a meteor that crashed to create the Nördlinger Ries Crater in Bohemia about 15 million years ago. Meteor crystals carry a different vibration than Earth crystals. If both cosmic and Earth-based crystals act like ancient computers, absorbing all the knowledge and information they are exposed to, then a meteor crystal opens you up to cosmic knowledge, whereas an Earth-based crystal opens you up to the more earthbound variety. Moldavite creates change in your life on a cosmic level, stimulating synchronicities (meaningful coincidences) and the downloading of spiritual knowledge. P.S. Moldavite can also slow down the body's aging process. Someone please create a Moldavite-based face serum, pronto!

Mystical Homework: Want to access the greater knowledge of the universe? Wear a Moldavite ring on your Jupiter/pointer finger, as in Vedic astrology, this finger represents expansion in our lives. Since it isn't originally from this planet, Moldavite carries the vibration of the cosmos, instead of the vibration of the earth. That's some power!

Crystal Affirmation: "I am expansive!"

31. Mookaite

AKA: "The Beauty Buzz"

The Look: A swirling blend of red, yellow, brown, taupe, tan, gold, and purple . . . kind of like a makeup palette

Where It Comes From: Australia

The "C Spot": 1st/Root, 2nd/Sacral, and 3rd/Solar Plexus Chakras

Why You Need It in Your Life: I hand this one out to every beauty industry person I meet, as it is known as the "Stone of Radiant Beauty." We all know that beauty is more than skin deep, and this stone helps

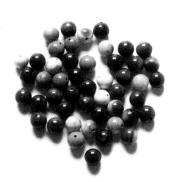

us to embody the traits of inner beauty, including self-worth, self-confidence, compassion, creativity, and intelligence.

Mystical Homework: Want to say thank you to the go-to beauty person (or people) in your life? This is a great gift for your favorite hair stylist/colorist, makeup artist, aesthetician, or manicurist.

Crystal Affirmation: "I am beautiful, inside and out."

32. Moonstone

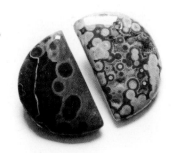

AKA: "Moon Goddess To-Go"

The Look: White and opalescent

Where It Comes From: Australia, Brazil, India, Madagascar, Mexico, Myanmar, Norway, Sri Lanka

The "C Spot": 2nd/Sacral Chakra

Why You Need It in Your Life: Moonstone honors the lunar goddess, and regulates feminine energies, childbirth, pregnancy, sensitivity, self-expression, love, desire, fertility, emotion, inner rhythms, and new beginnings. Historically, it has been used to provide protection during travel at night, under the light of the moon.

Mystical Homework: This is the ultimate fertility stone. If you are looking to get pregnant, keep Moonstone in close proximity. If you are already pregnant, bring this stone with you to Lamaze class, and into the delivery room to use as a "push stone" during labor.

Crystal Affirmation: "I love myself to the moon and back."

33. Ocean Jasper

AKA: "Chill the F*** Out"

The Look: A multicolored petri dish of blue, green, pink, and white circles, blobs, and other shapes

Where It Comes From: Madagascar

The "C Spot": 4th/Heart Chakra

Why You Need It in Your Life: Also known as Sea Jasper, this stone conveys the healing powers of the ocean. It's a watery stone that promotes peace, tranquility, cleanliness, letting go, and being present.

Mystical Homework: Take your Ocean Jasper with you to the beach at sunset. Stick your feet in the sand and wash your stone in the surf, while taking deep, calming breaths.

Crystal Affirmation: "I can chill the f*** out, dammit!"

34. Orange Calcite

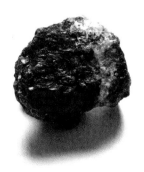

AKA: "B-12"

The Look: Orange

Where It Comes From: Mexico

The "C Spot": 2nd/Sacral Chakra

Why You Need It in Your Life: Orange Calcite is strongly associated with physical wellness and the physical body. It promotes physical, emotional, and mental balance so you can function at maximum capacity.

Mystical Homework: If you are feeling fatigued or have a case of the lazies, make a daily ritual of meditating with this stone, just like taking a vitamin.

Crystal Affirmation: "I am full of vitality."

35. Peacock Ore

AKA: "The Mystical Manifester"

The Look: All the colors of a peacock feather

Where It Comes From: Australia, Kazakhstan, United States, Zaire, Zimbabwe

The "C Spot": 7th/Crown Chakra

Why You Need It in Your Life: Peacock Ore works to manifest the mystical into physical existence in your life. Here are a few examples of how this could arise: You want to make friends with a psychic; you are looking to join a Moon Circle; you have "the gift" and are looking to call a teacher into your life. Peacock Ore also helps to turn on your psychic senses, and to keep you in a protective space while doing so.

Mystical Homework: Want to host a New Moon Ceremony? To form your Moon Circle, call in your high-vibe girl tribe, inviting those ladies closest to you who you believe would be open to a little spiritual enlightenment to join you on the day of the new moon. Mystical babes gather on the new moon because this is the best time in the moon cycle to call in and connect with the things we want in life. Don't forget the candles and snacks!

Crystal Affirmation: "I trust in my gifts."

36. Pink Botswana Agate

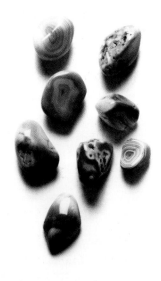

AKA: "Lonely Hearts Club"

The Look: Bands of pink and gray

Where It Comes From: Africa

The "C Spot": All

Why You Need It in Your Life: Pink Botswana Agate is the stone for you if you're in the middle of a major FML moment, have suffered a loss, or are struggling with emotional pain, loneliness, depression, grief, or destructive mental patterns. This stone deals with the heavies—it's about facing your sh*t (your "shadow") in a big way. By combating loneliness, grief, and depression, it ultimately makes room for joy.

Mystical Homework: If you are experiencing a time of loss or grief, this is a great stone to keep tucked away in your bra, close to your healing heart.

Crystal Affirmation: "I call in joy!!!"

37. Pink Moonstone

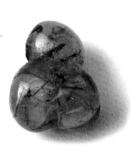

AKA: "The Hormone Slayer"

The Look: Pink or peach

Where It Comes From: Australia, Brazil, India, Germany, Sri Lanka, Madagascar, Mexico, Myanmar, Norway, Switzerland, Tanzania, United States

The "C Spot": 2nd//Sacral Chakra

Why You Need It in Your Life: Also known as Peach Moonstone, this one is for all the ladies out there dealing with hormone imbalances, mood swings, menstrual issues, fertility issues, or pregnancy. That's all of us at some point or another, right?

*Mystical Homework:*Wondering what to bring to a baby shower? Pink Moonstone is a great gift for your pregnant friends!

Crystal Affirmation: "I will recognize and honor all my feelings. Emotions are only temporary."

38. Prehnite

AKA: "The Magic Maker"

The Look: Green

Where It Comes From: Australia, Canada, China, Germany, France, Scotland, United States

The "C Spot": 4th/Heart Chakra and 6th/Third-Eye Chakra

Why You Need It in Your Life: Prehnite is known as the "Stone of Faerie Magic and Prophecy," and it's the official talisman of Freya, goddess of Nordic shamanism. With a calling card like that, you can only imagine what comes next: This stone assists with all the woo-woo stuff, including astral travel, dream work, tapping into past lives, communicating with the beyond, and boosting prophetic abilities.

Mystical Homework: If you are looking to enhance your fortune-telling skills and energize your personal tarot deck, keep a piece of Prehnite on top of your deck when it's not in use.

Crystal Affirmation: "I am enchanting."

39. Red Jasper

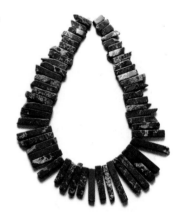

AKA: "The Triathlete"

The Look: Red, like Heinz ketchup

Where It Comes From: Australia, Brazil, Egypt, India, Indonesia, Kazakhstan, Madagascar, Russia, Uruguay, United States, Venezuela

The "C Spot": 2nd/Sacral Chakra

Why You Need It in Your Life: Known as the "Stone of Endurance" and used to stimulate chi/prana/life force, Red Jasper promotes physical strength, stamina, and energy, as well as mental determination and focus.

Mystical Homework: Train for a marathon with a piece of Red Jasper in your sports bra.

Crystal Affirmation: "Only 26.2 more miles to go!"

40. Rhodonite

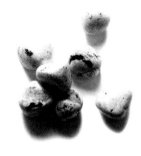

AKA: "The Heartbreak Healer"

The Look: Pink and black

Where It Comes From: Australia, Brazil, Canada, England, Peru, Russia, Sweden, United States

The "C Spot": 4th/Heart Chakra

Why You Need It in Your Life: Been through the emotional ringer? Rhodonite is like energetic first-aid for the heart. It heals emotional trauma, past and present, that may be the result of unrequited or obsessive love, codependent love and jealousy, or grief and loss over failed relationships.

Mystical Homework: Nurture a broken heart by sticking a small piece of Rhodonite in your bra, and keeping it close to your heart and your Heart Chakra.

Crystal Affirmation: "I will recover and heal."

41. Sardonyx

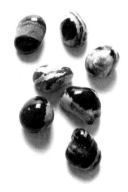

AKA: "The Résumé Builder"

The Look: Earth tones alternating with bands of white

Where It Comes From: Australia, Brazil, China, India, South Africa, Russia, Ukraine, United States

The "C Spot": 1st/Root Chakra

Why You Need It in Your Life: This is the stone of first impressions. It helps you manifest the characteristics that you want to embody and that you want people to see in you upon first meeting. It's the perfect stone for interviews! Sardonyx builds character, is great for confidence and positive attitude, and helps you digest information with greater understanding.

Mystical Homework: Meditate with this stone to call in your dream job.

Crystal Affirmation: "I am able."

42. Scolecite

AKA: "The Stepping Stone"

The Look: White

Where It Comes From: Antarctica, Australia, Austria, Brazil, Bulgaria, Canada, Chile, Czechoslovakia, England, Ethiopia, France, Germany, Greenland, Hungary, Iceland, Italy, India, Japan, Mexico, Mozambique, Nicaragua, Peru, Poland, Scotland, South Africa, Sweden, Switzerland, Taiwan, United States, Yugoslavia

The "C Spot": 6th/Third-Eye Chakra

Why You Need It in Your Life: Also known as a "connectivity crystal," this stone helps us get from point A to point B. It helps us to connect, network, work in unison, and embody good old team spirit with whomever we call our tribe.

Mystical Homework: Keep on your desk at work.

Crystal Affirmation: "I am a conductor for change."

43. Serpentine

AKA: "The Goddess Kali"

The Look: Green with splashes of white or blue

Where It Comes From: Afghanistan, Austria, Canada, France, Greece, Italy, Korea, Myanmar, New Zealand, Norway, Russia

The "C Spot": 1st/Root Chakra

Why You Need It in Your Life: This stone helps us with renewal, so we can shed our skin, one layer at a time, in order to keep growing. This stone reminds me of the Hindu goddess Kali, known as the "Great Destroyer," who shakes things up and destroys with the intention to create something new, and more aligned with our personal path.

Mystical Homework: Looking to shed a few things in your life that no longer serve your highest and greatest good? Embrace your inner snake! Make a list of all the people, things, and situations in your life that feel like last season's trends, and while meditating, slither down your shed list. Hold this stone and imagine letting go of each item, and picture the freedom this new space will bring into your life.

Crystal Affirmation: "I will allow what doesn't serve me to fall away . . . without fighting it."

44. Shaman Quartz

AKA: "The Mercurial Cure"

The Look: Colorless with green, red, yellow, or rutile inclusions

Where It Comes From: Brazil

The "C Spot": 7th/Crown Chakra

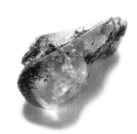

Why You Need It in Your Life: Known alternately as Scenic Quartz, Landscape Quartz, Garden Quartz, Lodolite, and Shaman Dream Quartz, this is your go-to stone when Mercury is in retrograde! The expression "Mercury in retrograde" refers to this planet being in apparent (as opposed to actual) motion due to the relative positions of Mercury and Earth, and how they are moving around the sun. Mercury governs communication, negotiations, shipping, travel, and transportation, and when it's in retrograde, we can literally feel a shift in the aforementioned categories. Many people experience this time as feeling chaotic. However, we should recognize that it also highlights (sometimes in big flashing lights) the things that are not working for us. Shaman Quartz helps us to sort through this turmoil, in order to make way for personal reflection and address what needs tending to in our lives.

Mystical Homework: To help ease the universal and unavoidable sway of Mercury when it goes retro, keep this stone in your purse during the duration of this three- to four-week cycle, which happens several times a year. And *do not* sign any contracts when Merc goes retro!

Crystal Affirmation: "I glide through the chaos with a sense of humor."

45. Snowflake Obsidian

AKA: "Emotional Baggage, Be Gone!"
The Look: Black with whitish-gray freckles
Where It Comes From: Any place with high amounts of volcanic activity, including Argentina, Armenia, Azerbaijan, Australia, Canada, Chile, Georgia, Greece, El Salvador, Guatemala, Iceland, Italy, Japan, Kenya, Mexico, New Zealand, Papua New Guinea, Peru, Scotland, Turkey, United States

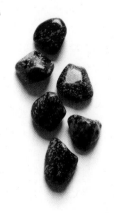

The "C Spot": 1st/Root Chakra

Why You Need It in Your Life: Snowflake Obsidian helps us to honor and learn from the tough life lessons (aka f***-ups) that we all face, and to move on from them. It's time to put those failures and rough spots behind us.

Mystical Homework: Take a look at the old, unhealthy emotional patterns that seem to reappear in your life. Everyone has a few. If you're not sure what they are, try filling in the blank: "Every time I _____, I become a screaming, crying, ice cream–eating, drama-mama hot mess." Take the word or phrase you used to fill in the blank and write it down on a piece of paper, then put a piece of Snowflake Obsidian on top of it. Make it a practice to look at what you've written on this piece of paper every day until you feel yourself starting to release that old, unhealthy emotional pattern.

Crystal Affirmation: "I do not allow old emotional patterns to dictate my future actions."

46. Sodalite

AKA: "Nothing But the Truth"

The Look: Royal blue with white striations

Where It Comes From: Brazil, Bolivia, Canada, Greenland, Portugal, Romania, Russia, United States

The "C Spot": 5th/Throat Chakra

Why You Need It in Your Life: Call on Sodalite, the "Poet's Stone," if you are having trouble speaking the truth, seeing the truth within a situation, or seeing both sides of a situation with an objective eye. This communication-

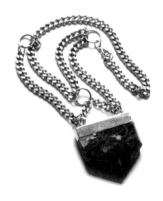

enhancing stone is great for writers, those who do a lot of public speaking, and anyone who tends to get defensive or overly sensitive in conversations.

Mystical Homework: Cat got your tongue? We all experience occasional moments of speechlessness, where we're afraid to say what's on our minds or don't know how to respond to something that has been said to us. Sodalite is the perfect stone to wear around your neck in situations where you may find yourself at a loss for words—at a networking event, a job interview, or when you have something tough to say to someone.

Crystal Affirmation: "I speak my truth, with love, no matter what."

47. Spinel

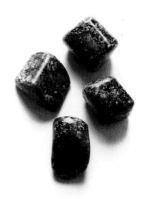

AKA: "The Workaholic's Crown Jewel"

The Look: Various colors, including black, white, pink, yellow, blue, green, peach, red, and purple

Where It Comes From: Australia, Brazil, Cambodia, Kenya, Myanmar, Madagascar, Nepal, Nigeria, Sri Lanka, Tanzania, Thailand, United States, Vietnam

The "C Spot": All

Why You Need It in Your Life: Some of the most famous jewels in the world are Spinels, and you can find them among the crown jewels of many royal households. Spinel is a great stone for workaholics and entrepreneurs because it helps to release stress and worry, breathe fresh air into work endeavors, and replenish depleted energy from an overly vigorous work life.

Mystical Homework: Place Spinel on your desk, put your out-of-office on, and take a mental health day! Set aside this time to clear your headspace, make room for fresh perspectives, and rejuvenate the body.

Crystal Affirmation: "I can take a day off. It's good for my sanity!"

48. Sugilite

AKA: "The Shield"

The Look: Anna Sui purple

Where It Comes From: Australia, Canada, Italy, India, South Africa

The "C Spot": 7th/Crown Chakra

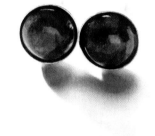

Why You Need It in Your Life: Sugilite is one of the best crystals for those who are highly sensitive, also known as empaths or HSPs (highly sensitive people). It provides an energetic shield from people, places, and things in your environment. Sugilite is also known as the "Healer's Stone" because it enhances healing on a mental, physical, emotional, and spiritual level. Due to its high Manganese content, this stone also excels at soothing headaches.

Mystical Homework: If you are a sufferer of migraines, try wearing Sugilite earrings for relief. This keeps the gems in close proximity to the afflicted area.

Crystal Affirmation: "I am safe."

49. Super Seven

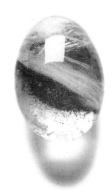

AKA: "The Khaleesi"

The Look: Transparent or translucent and filled with inclusions of confetti-like metallic pieces in hues of gold, orange, pink, and purple

Where It Comes From: Brazil

The "C Spot": All

Why You Need It in Your Life: This is a crystal that actually contains seven different materials: Amethyst, Cacoxenite, Clear Quartz, Goethite, Lepidocrocite, Rutile, and Smoky Quartz. It's basically six crystals sandwiched inside an "amplifier" crystal. The Super Seven crystal is like an eat-your-fire-for-breakfast girl boss who still manages to remain charming and stylish, with not a hair out of place. Her supernatural dance card includes enhancing psychic abilities such as clairvoyance, clairaudience, telepathy, telekinesis, channeling, chatting with Spirit Guides, seeing auras, spiritual grounding and growth, and psychic protection. P.S. This super stone never needs cleansing or recharging . . . so she cleans up after herself, too!

Mystical Homework: Keep in mind that her girlish charm packs a punch. So, after purchasing, slowly integrate Super Seven into your crystal practice. Keep it in your space before wearing it, for example.

Crystal Affirmation: "I am the Mother of Dragons."

50. Unakite

AKA: "Unity, Baby"

The Look: Grass green and salmon pink

Where It Comes From: South Africa, Switzerland, United States

The "C Spot": 5th/Throat Chakra

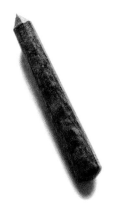

Why You Need It in Your Life: Unakite aligns body and spirit. It's a spiritually grounding stone, meaning that it helps you to connect with your Spirit Guides while still keeping your feet firmly planted in reality. It can also help with working through tough emotions like confusion, depression, and anxiety.

Mystical Homework: Has our current political climate, along with recent social, economic, and global events got you down? Hold this stone and breathe, breathe, breathe.

Crystal Affirmation: "I call in alignment."

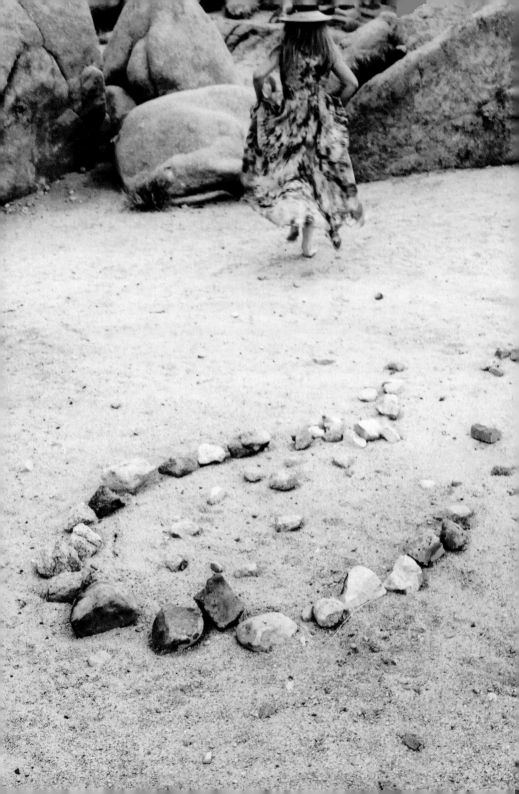

5

ROCK IT! CRYSTALS IN EVERY AREA OF YOUR LIFE

For the great doesn't happen through impulse alone and is a succession of little things that are brought together.

–VINCENT VAN GOGH

SPIRITUAL HYGIENE: CLEANSING YOUR CRYSTALS

We care for our bodies with exercise, healthy diet, skincare, and plenty of sleep. Why wouldn't we care for the *energy* surrounding our bodies in a similar way? This is where spiritual hygiene comes in. As we've discussed, crystals receive, store, and transmit energy. By the time you bring your stone home, it will have picked up energy from each person and place it has been in contact with. This accumulated energy may be described as dense, stale, negative or simply just not "yours"—and if you've been working with a stone for a while, these collected vibes may have actually come from you! So it's important to regularly "cleanse" and energetically recharge your crystals. It's like washing your face daily to remove dirt and debris!

There are many ways to cleanse your crystals, in order to allow them to reset, rebalance, and function at their optimum frequency. All methods involve working with the healing powers of Mother Nature and the Five Elements: aether (the element that encompasses the cosmos, all celestial bodies—it is known as the subtlest element, and essentially means space), air, earth, fire, and water. Some crystal cleansing methods are better for high-vibration stones. Some methods aren't right for crystals that are soft or porous, or that contain metals. And some crystals are actually self-cleaning. So be informed before you begin!

Pre-Cleanse Tips

- **SET AN INTENTION:** Like all rituals, crystal cleansing is ultimately about intention. Make sure you are in a positive mood while cleaning your crystals, and if you have a specific purpose in mind for a stone, mentally share that intent with the stone as you clean it. In your mind's eye, visualize the unwanted energy being released from the crystal and sent back to the earth to be mulched for positivity. Send the universe a mental thank-you note when done to close your cleansing ritual.

- **CLEANSE ON THE FULL MOON:** I like to cleanse my stones monthly on the full moon, when its energy is the strongest, in order to embrace the moon's energy to enhance my intentions.

- **DON'T SHARE YOUR CRYSTALS!** I know, it sounds stingy, but don't let others touch your crystals once they are attuned to you. Would you

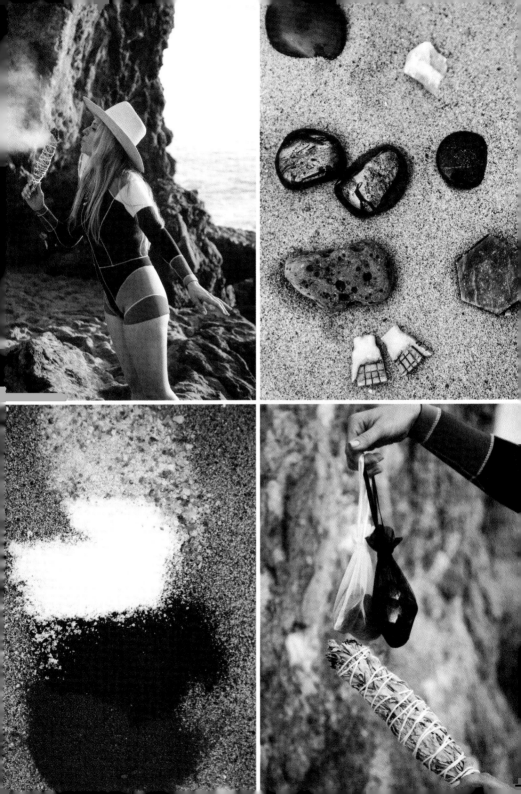

share your lipstick, mascara, or toothbrush? It's the same thing!

- **DRESS FOR THE OCCASION:** Wear black. Why? Traditionally, shamans wear black when performing cleansing rites and rituals like house clearings and exorcisms. They believe that black deflects bad vibes and makes them "invisible" to the spirits present. And practically speaking, if you are burning lit herbs to clear your crystals (which we'll get into later), you don't want to ruin your outfit.

HOW TO CLEAN YOUR STONES

There are many differing approaches to cleansing stones, but I am introducing you to the top methods I've learned from my mentors, stemming from various esoteric traditions. Borrow the practices here that resonate most strongly with you and that are the most practical for your lifestyle.

1. *Start digging:* Bury your crystals in dirt or sand in your backyard. Returning them to the earth cleanses them and allows them to recharge with the vibration of the earth. I leave them buried for anywhere between 48 hours and an entire moon cycle (about a month). Make sure to mark where your crystals are buried so that you can retrieve them later. If you are a city-dweller, bury your stones in a potted houseplant.

2. *H_2O, go!*: Place your crystals in a clean, glass container and let them soak overnight in water. I recommend using mineral water, spring water, or purified water over tap water. You can also submerge your crystal in a bowl of fresh rainwater, or hold it in a lake or stream for five to ten minutes while visualizing any negativity being washed away by the water.

3. *Get salty:* Washing crystals in salt water is also great because salt absorbs and purifies unwanted energies. You can visit the beach or make salt water at home. Use a clean glass container, and be

sure not to use too much salt, as undissolved salt can scratch some stones. A general rule of thumb is to use 1 to 2 tablespoons salt for every 8 ounces water. Let your stones soak for at least 24 hours, and after removing them from the salt water, rinse them in fresh water to remove any salt residue.

4. *Hold the H_2O!:* Some crystals disintegrate when wet or don't react well to being immersed in salt water. You should only cleanse with water/salt water when stones measure 7 or above (Quartz or harder) on the Mohs' scale of mineral hardness. Google the Mohs' scale and read up on whether this method is safe for your stones. If not, you can let them sit in a bowl of coarse sea salt, or even table salt, for 24 to 48 hours.

5. *I'll take a side of rice, please:* Place your crystal in a container (preferably glass) of brown rice, cover completely, and leave overnight. The rice will absorb unwanted bad vibes from the stones. Make sure to dispose of the rice after this method.

6. *Bathe in moonlight:* Lunar energy helps cleanse and charge stones. The moon's light is brightest and energetically strongest during the full moon, but if your schedule is jam-packed on the actual full moon, you can also work with the energy 24 hours prior to and 24 hours after the actual full moon. If you are dealing with a crystal that fades or that doesn't like light (see the list on page 153), be sure to bring it back inside before the sun comes up. Put this crystal on a glass or ceramic plate and leave it to sit out overnight on your deck, fire escape, in your backyard, etc. Let the cosmos do the rest.

7. *Burn, baby, burn:* Burn sage and run your crystal through the smoke. In addition to the ritual cleansing of a space, scientists have observed that sage can also clear up to 94 percent of airborne bacteria in a space—it's powerful stuff. Other qualities believed to be associated with the burning of sage are increased wisdom, clarity, and spiritual awareness. Here are the basics for cleansing, or "smudging," with sage:

- You are lighting something on fire, so the right container is key. Traditionally, abalone shells have been used to hold burning sage, but a glass or ceramic bowl will work, too.

- Once finished, the best way to extinguish your smudge stick is by pressing the burning surface firmly against a fireproof bowl or stone, or in dirt or sand, until smoke no longer rises. Don't use water to extinguish the hot embers—it will ruin the tip of the stick and makes it harder to light the next time.

- Once you are done, make triple sure that every bit of fire and smoke has been extinguished and rest the remaining sage in the shell or nonflammable container until you are ready to use it again.

- Have an exit strategy. Before you light up, remember to open a door or a window so the unwanted energy you are trying to clear out will have a path of escape. For escorting out unwanted energy, I like to employ the mantra, "Any energy that is not mine or of my highest and greatest good, get the f*** out, with love."

- If you don't like the smell of sage, you can also employ other sacred materials in smudging, like copal (a type of tree resin) or palo santo wood.

8. *Firedancer:* Scientifically and spiritually speaking, fire is the most transformative of all the elements. Traditionally, shamans use fire to cleanse their crystals before and after performing an "extraction" (a process similar to an exorcism that releases extremely heavy, stuck, or unwanted energy from a person's physical body). Since extraction is a very intense type of energy work, shamans need to pull out the big guns and run their crystals though an open flame before and after to make sure they are energetically spotless. I advise people to use this technique if they feel like they just can't get a crystal clean through one of the other techniques mentioned. You don't need access to a fireplace or

camp-style bonfire—you can do this at home on your deck or in your backyard. And remember to pull your hair back before trying this super-shaman-y maneuver! You will need:

- A disposable foil baking dish or heat-safe glass bowl
- Epsom salts
- Isopropyl rubbing alcohol
- A long-reach lighter or long-stemmed matches
- Something to quickly extinguish the fire

Place 1/4 cup of Epsom salts into your heat-safe container. (If you're using a bowl, make sure the surface beneath the bowl will not be damaged by heat). Pour rubbing alcohol onto the Epsom salts in a ratio of about 2:1 Epsom salts to alcohol. You want the salts to be damp, but not soaked. If you try to light the salts and the flame burns weakly, you've added too little alcohol.

When you're ready to begin, touch the flame to the salt. It will instantly ignite. You want a mostly blue flame with a hint of yellow. If your flame is mostly yellow, you have put too much alcohol into the mix. Add a little more salt to correct. This type of burning doesn't create smoke or smells, so you can do it indoors, with a door or window open to allow negative energy to leave the space.

Run your crystal back and forth through the flame in a figure-eight motion. In your mind's eye, envision the blue flame eating up all the unwanted energy, and recite any mantra or invocation you feel called to. Once finished, smother the flames with a pot lid, and after the salts cool down, please discard them responsibly, either in the toilet or by burying them deeply in the earth, as Epsom salts can give animals diarrhea and other health problems if ingested.

If you are not feeling this brave, but want to try to work with the element of fire, use a candle flame to start.

9. ***Sun bathing:*** Leave your crystals out in direct sunlight for a duration that feels right to you—normally one day does the trick. Remember, some crystals do not like light, and will fade or become brittle after exposure to direct UV rays. If you live in an extremely hot place with strong sunlight, put crystals out only early in the morning or late in the afternoon when the sun's rays aren't as strong, to ensure the crystals don't crack or explode in the intense heat.

10. ***Hot hands:*** If you or someone you know is Reiki attuned, you can clear your crystals with Reiki. Hold your crystal in your hands, or hover your cupped hands over the crystal, and breathe deeply. While focusing on your breath, try to feel the positive energies of the stone. Visualize universal, healing light filling the stone until all negativity has been dissolved. Set an intention that all negative energies be removed from the stone. When you intuitively feel that the stone has been cleared, you can stop the visualization.

11. ***Breathwork it!:*** If you have ever experienced a shamanic healing, you may have seen the shaman forcefully breathe over the crystals after the work is done. This is a quick and easily accessible way to remove unwanted energy.

12. ***Crystal on crystal:*** To draw out impurities, place your crystal on top of a larger crystal cluster like Clear Quartz, Citrine, or Amethyst. You can also use a large, flat piece of self-cleansing Selenite and place your crystals like ants on a log on top of it. Let the crystals sit for 24 hours to draw out impurities.

13. ***Good vibrations:*** You can use *tingsha* bells, tuning forks, Peruvian brass bells, gongs, chimes, or a crystal or metal singing bowl to send cleansing sound vibrations into your crystal for 2 to 5 minutes. Be careful about placing your crystals within an actual singing bowl, as the intense vibration of the bowl may chip fragile stones.

14. ***Essences and sprays:*** Use cleansing essential oils like juniper, pine, or sage. Heat them in a burner or vaporizer and then pass your crystals through the vapor that's given off. You can also place a few drops of an essence in a bowl of water and then soak your crystals, or you can spray them with a solution of water mixed with 5 to 7 drops of the essence in a small spray bottle or plant mister. I use Paper Crane Apothecary sprays as my go-tos when traveling! (You'll hear more from the founder later in the book.)

Self-Cleansing Crystals: Amethyst, Azeztulite, Black Tourmaline, Citrine, Kyanite, Smoky Quartz, Selenite

Personally, I still clean all my crystals, self-cleansing or not, because I believe they benefit from the care and maintenance.

HOT TIP: *Clear Quartz and Carnelian can cleanse other stones as well but will likely need to be cleansed when done.*

Crystals That Cannot Get Wet: Amber, Angelite, Azurite, Celestite, Calcite, Fire Opal, Fluorite, Kyanite, Kunzite, Moonstone, Turquoise, Rhodochrosite, and Selenite

HOT TIP: *Many stones that end in "–ite" are not water-friendly.*

Crystals That Fade or Crack in the Sun: Aventurine, Amethyst, Aquamarine, Beryl, Citrine, Chrysocolla, Fluorite, Kunzite, Rose Quartz, Sapphire, Smoky Quartz. Amber and Opal can become brittle from the sun, causing them to crack, chip, or split. Fluorite is the only crystal on the planet to have *two* internal lattice structures (every other crystal has only one). Sunlight breaks down one of those structures, causing Fluorite to shatter easily.

HOW OFTEN SHOULD CRYSTALS BE CLEANSED?

Altar: Crystals that live on altars should be cleaned on average once a month. I make it a ritual to completely dismantle my altar every new and full moon. I physically clean the surface with earth-friendly cleaning products and then rearrange all my crystals, tarot cards, talismans etc.

Spatial: If you've had your space gridded by a shaman or fêng shui practitioner, please consult them on this. I like to recharge the crystals that sit in the corners of my home about once a year around an event like spring cleaning.

Wearable: This includes jewelry, and the crystals you squirrel away in your bra. If you wear a crystal or meditate with it daily, it should be cleaned once a week. If someone touches your crystal, take it off and stick it in a cotton or velvet pouch until you can clean it.

RE-UPPING YOUR CRYSTAL MOJO: HOW TO CHARGE YOUR CRYSTALS

Cleansing your stones is the first step. Your next order of business is to "charge" or energize your crystals in order to reinforce your connection with them, whether you are working with newly acquired stones or stones you have had for a long time. A crystal is a bit like a battery: It vibrates at a certain frequency, and when you use it, it discharges positive energy into your body. This is why people report feeling tingles, zaps, jolts, or heat in their body when wearing or handling a crystal; the energy of our body is merging with that of the crystal. But it will eventually run out of juice and need to be recharged. Here are the methods I rely on for recharging crystals:

- **SLEEPING WITH, MEDITATING WITH, AND HANDLING YOUR CRYSTALS:** Another great place to start when energizing your crystals is to simply spend time "getting to know each other" by sleeping with them at your bedside, meditating with them, or just handling them.

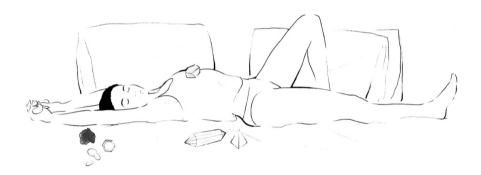

- **CRYSTAL DEDICATION RITUAL:** In a quiet setting, hold your crystal. Start by taking a few deep breaths with your eyes closed to relax your breathing. Notice how you are feeling, what the stone feels like in your hand, and what your energy feels like together. Then either think or say aloud a dedication to connect your personal energy with your crystal. Here are examples of what your dedication might be:

"I intend for our work together to be . . ."

"I accept this gift from the Universe, and I ask my crystal to . . ."

"With love, gratitude, and purest intentions, I call in . . ."

- BATHING IN MOONLIGHT: I recommend energizing your crystals monthly under the light of the full moon. Leave your crystal out in the moonlight under the same conditions mentioned in the crystal clearing section.

- BATHING IN SUNLIGHT: Leave your crystal out in direct sunlight under the same conditions mentioned in the crystal clearing section.

- SOUND BATHING: This one is extra credit. Stick a crystal inside a crystal or metal singing bowl, or, if the crystal is fragile, place it 2 to 4 inches away from the singing bowl. Hold the singing bowl in the palm of your left hand, grasp the mallet in your right hand, and gently tap it against the side of the bowl to "warm" it. Keeping even pressure, rub the mallet clockwise around the outside edge of the bowl. Keep the mallet facing up and down (north and south) while moving your arm (not your wrist) like you are stirring a pot of soup. Apply pressure evenly, as the friction from the mallet against the rim of the bowl is what produces vibrations and creates sound.

HOW LONG WILL A CRYSTAL BE IN MY LIFE?

My personal practice is to keep working with a crystal until I get a sign that our time together is over, meaning that the crystal cracks, chips, breaks in half, shatters, or explodes, or I just feel that our work together is done. Some believe that if a crystal cracks into two perfect halves, it's a sign that your crystal needs to move on to someone else, and you should either keep one half and give the other to someone in your life who needs it, or give both halves to two people who need them more than you do.

Sometimes your crystal will let you know loud and clear that it has served its energetic purpose. I was once standing on a street corner in New York City and looked down to find that the bottom half of the Black Agate I always wore around my neck was lying on the pavement. Back then I had no idea what I was doing, and I loved this piece so much that I decided to superglue it back together (can you imagine?). The next day I found myself standing on the same street corner, and when I reached down to clutch my Agate, I discovered it had cracked again, below the glue line. This crystal had sent me a clear message that it was time to part ways—twice!

I have heard of people who choose to keep working with cracked stones, but this is not my personal practice. If you do decide to keep a cracked stone, bear in mind that the energy that caused it to crack was intense, and this may have temporarily altered the crystal's normal vibrational frequency. It takes a crystal some time to heal from this trauma, just like a broken bone takes time to heal. If you choose to keep a broken crystal, give it a little vacay before you start using it again, and be sure to cleanse it before use.

ASPIRING HEALERS, PLEASE NOTE: *If a crystal breaks during any healing application, it should never be used again for a healing treatment or anything else. The crystal broke because it absorbed unwanted energy that came out of someone's body, and it is time to put it to rest.*

THANK YOU FOR YOUR SERVICE

Wondering what to do with a broken crystal? Since the earth absorbs and recycles both energy and matter, I return a cracked crystal to the elements by burying it in the woods or releasing it into a body of water. Before I do this, I always "deprogram" my crystal by thanking it for working with me and asking for my energy to be removed from it.

ALTAR'D STATES

Altar building is a practice in many spiritual traditions, spanning all ancient faiths from Buddhism to Christianity to Judaism to Paganism. An altar is any structure upon which offerings are made for a specific occasion/reason, and altars can be dedicated to many purposes, from honoring ancestors and universal unseen forces we believe are protecting and guiding us to manifesting situations and showing gratitude to something. For thousands of years, altars have been built in churches and temples, on sacred grounds and shrines, and in other places of worship. I view altars as a kind of common meeting point for all faiths and traditions.

A personal crystal altar does not have to be elaborate or fancy. I like to look at altars as an extension of who we are, and think of them as an endlessly evolving, living, breathing organism. It should simply be a special place to call your own, a quiet place for reflection, focus, and prayer, for thinking positive thoughts, manifesting your desires, and honoring who and what is important to you. And you can turn just about any place in your home or garden into your own sacred space for a crystal altar.

Altar Building, Step by Step

1. *Location, location, location:* Find a spot that suits your lifestyle, budget, and space. You don't need to dedicate an entire room in your house to your altar—all you need is a cozy corner where you already tend to feel comfortable, happy, and inspired. An altar can be located on a bookshelf, in a walk-in closet, on a fire escape, on your makeup vanity table, among your houseplants, on a desk or credenza, or in your backyard garden. Just follow your heart and intuition and find a place that feels right to you. You may want to have one altar in a central location in your home, or several smaller altars around your space, each dedicated to a different endeavor.

P.S.: *Make sure to choose a place for your altar that is out of reach for children or animals who might get curious about its contents or knock things over.*

EXTRA CREDIT: *Work with a fêng shui practitioner to map out the energy of your space on a bagua chart, for advice on the best place for your altar.*

2. ***Clear the decks:*** Once you have your location, clear away any items that don't make sense from around the chosen space. Your altar is the gateway for new ideas, desires, and intentions to emerge and manifest, and it's important to honor the space you have chosen by making it clean and beautiful. Go Kondo on your space, move furniture, and don't forget the Mrs. Meyer's and the Dyson before you set up your crystals.

3. ***Set an intention:*** Decide on an intention for your altar, depending on what you want to devote your time and energy to. Common intentions for altars include: Love, Money, Manifestation, Meditation, Family Matters/Honoring Ancestors, Career Issues, Inspiration/Creativity, Expressing Gratitude, and Friendship.

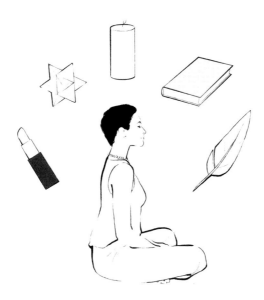

Building a Love Altar

I like to get creative with my clients when it comes to altar building. Recently I was working with a client who wanted to call new love and sexual experiences into her life. First we located the Relationships direction on her fêng shui *bagua* chart, and found the corresponding location in her home. Then we placed a shiny, red lacquer tray in this spot and placed the following items on her altar:

- Rose Quartz, the stone of self-love and love of others
- Clear Quartz, an amplifier stone
- Agent Provocateur lingerie
- Sex toys
- Chocolate
- Red and pink roses
- Red and pink candles
- A list of the qualities that she would like in a partner
- A rose oil–burning diffuser
- A picture of a couple on a beach in Bali
- Other miscellaneous personal items that symbolized love, sex, intimacy, and a healthy relationship to her

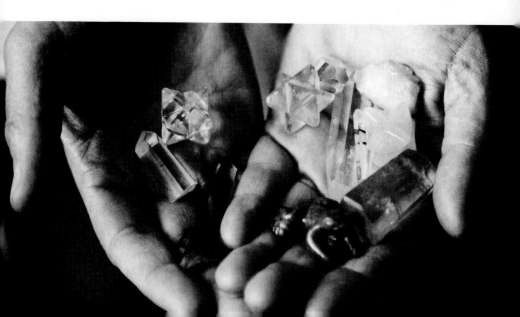

Building a Money Altar

I was working with a client who wanted to call monetary abundance into her life, so we first located her Success direction on her fêng shui *bagua* chart, then moved her desk to that area. Next we cleared an area for the altar on her desk and placed the following items on it:

- A crisp stack of one hundred $1 bills, with a piece of Citrine (the "Merchant's Stone" of abundance and personal power) on top
- A small crystal grid made with Citrine, Jade, Green Aventurine, Iron Pyrite, and Clear Quartz, for manifesting wealth (see the section on Crystal Gridding later in this chapter)
- My client was having trouble speaking her truth when it came to money, so I had her make a written list of everything she wanted to manifest with regards to money and her personal power. We put a piece of Lapis Lazuli with streaks of Iron Pyrite in it on top of the written list (since Lapis Lazuli is the "Stone of Communication" and Iron Pyrite is the "High Manifester").
- From a tarot reading, we also determined that my client had money trauma circulating from a past life, so we took the tarot card that represented this from our reading, and placed Hypersthene and Apache Tears on top of the card. (Apache Tears deals with grief, and Hypersthene encourages one to be less judgmental, promotes positive thinking, and works within the realm of past-life traumas.)
- A fêng shui money tree, also known as *Pachira aquatica*. Chinese legend states that the money tree can bring money and fortune to those who care for it, and that it's a symbol of affluence.
- A picture of what she envisioned her new office space to look like
- Other gold and green items

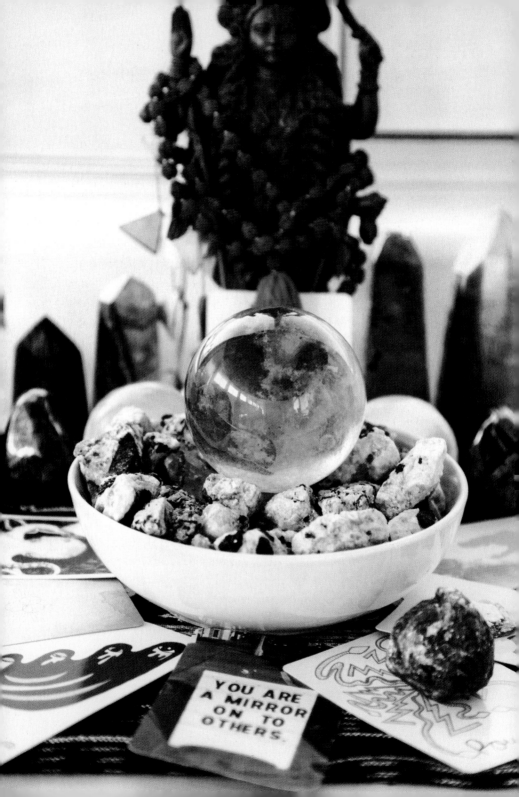

Building a Manifestation Altar

One of the most common questions I get asked is "How do I manifest _____?" My answer is that I believe in the law of attraction: You create your reality with your thoughts, words, and actions. Energy attracts energy, and you attract people, places, things, and experiences that are in vibrational harmony with your current and dominant frequency. Every aspect of your life, from the Benjamins in your bank account to your physical health to the quality of your relationships, is a reflection of the energy you are putting out there, positive or negative. And you can learn to work with energy! An intention altar is a great place to start learning how to move energy, and you don't have to be a quantum physicist or shaman to do it.

Items for building your manifestation altar:

- Iron Pyrite (high manifester) + Clear Quartz (amplifier) + a crystal that embodies what you are trying to call into your life (refer to the Top 20 Stones list, page 59, and Encyclopedia of Crystals, page 109)
- Manifestation list
- Vision board or chosen photo of what your end game looks like
- Items that represent what you are trying to call into your life. For example, if you are planning to go back to school, or simply want to call wisdom into your life, place books by people you admire or on the subjects you are interested in on your altar.

1. ***Find your altar style:*** This is the fun part, just like putting together an outfit. Remember, there are no "right" or "wrong" items for your altar. Trust in your intuition and choose what resonates with you by asking yourself the following questions:

   - ARE YOU CLASSIC? Choose a few key items that will never go out of style to anchor your altar, with a few interchangeable accessories.
   - ARE YOU TRENDY? If your mood changes like the weather, it's probably best to use items that have an expiration date like fresh-cut flowers, chocolate, and fruit.
   - ARE YOU A PEACOCK? Your altar may reflect this with lots of sparkly, over-the-top statement pieces all partying together.
   - ARE YOU A MINIMALIST? Keep your altar clean, simple, and basic with a few choice crystals and other items that inspire you.
   - ARE YOU EXOTIC OR BOHEMIAN? Every item on your altar will likely have a story from your world travels.
   - ARE YOU TRADITIONAL? Perhaps you're open to this whole altar/ moon circle/crystal stuff, but grew up in a traditionally religious household. Incorporate some traditional items that you're comfortable with, like candles, rosary beads, or a Bible.

   Once you've determined your "altar style," accessorize with some of the following items in addition to your crystals:

   - Candles, lamps, Christmas lights
   - Jewelry, *mala* beads, trinkets, and talismans
   - Tarot cards
   - Bowl of water or metal cubes and pyramids, as these are conductors for communicating with the spirit world

- The written word: spiritual or inspirational books; poems and song lyrics; greeting cards; thank-you notes; "I AM" statements; manifestation lists
- Photos of deities, family, friends, people you admire, and spiritual leaders
- Elements from nature: incense, flowers, fruit, potted plants, salt, sacred herbs, seashells, feathers
- Bells, chimes, sound bowls, tuning forks

2. *Charge your altar with good vibes:* When you feel that your altar is complete, set aside a few minutes to bless the space, invite good energy in, and ask for protection and inspiration from your Spirit Guides. Light a candle, burn some sage, pray, or just say, "Spirit Guides, life is a total sh*tstorm right now. I'm feeling lost and could really use your guidance—like, right f***ing now." Been there, done that. And it works!

3. *Visitation rites:* Your altar is much more than a decorative feature in your space. It's important to develop a daily, weekly, or monthly ritual for interacting with your altar. Develop a practice that works with your lifestyle, and make sure it's enjoyable and inviting, a ceremony full of rituals that send a message to the universe that you are committed to your intentions.

4. *Ritual reset:* On every new and full moon, I like to "reset" my altar to bring in new energy. So every fifteen days or so, I take everything off my altar, clean the items with cleaning products, and burn sacred herbs (with the windows open). All tarot cards, crystals, pictures, manifestation lists, etc., get completely rearranged (and I burn any tarot cards that represent old messages I have worked through). You can choose to reset your altar daily, weekly, monthly, or seasonally.

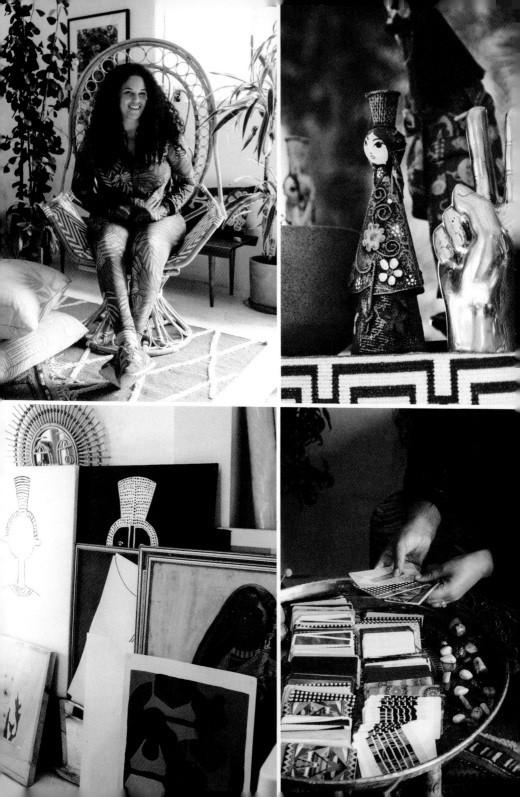

The Jungalow: Justina Blakeney

JUSTINA IS A DESIGNER, ARTIST, AND AUTHOR who believes creativity is the key to an amazing home, and you can see it oozing out of the pores of her LA headquarters. Upon entering "The Jungalow," I was greeted by furniture, rugs, pillows, plants, wallpaper, bedding, stationery, patterns, colors, and of course a collection of crystals. This *New York Times*–bestselling author has written six books on the subject, so I knew I had come to the right place to talk crystals with the High Priestess of bohemian environments.

How did you get into crystals?

I've loved them my whole life. A great-uncle who was an artist, for whom I am named, died right before I was born, and he bequeathed my sister and me his rock collection. He foraged for Turquoise and Coral and used it in his jewelry designs. I liked the feeling of holding crystals in my hands, as I remember feeling there was something very magical about them. My big love is indoor plants; they are an organic way to grow energies within the home. While researching for my most recent book, *The New Bohemians Handbook,* I learned more about the magic of crystals, and it became clear to me that the energies they can bring into the home are similar to plants, so that was the connection for me. I

intuitively feel the health benefits of crystals. I know when I am around them that they instill a sense of wonder and adventure in me.

How do you use crystals in your signature design formula?

Placement and function of crystals are key when I am decorating. I make suggestions on how to use them within the space in my book *Décor Magic.* I am a spiritual yet rational person. I am a mind-over-matter person, and if you believe it works, then it will work. Having a repeated energetic experience with certain crystals over and over provides rational meaning to me. I find that infusing fêng shui and plants with crystals is a spiritual way to interact with your home. I like the idea of them being magic and meaning different things to different people. When I am decorating for myself, I like to experiment with placement of crystals with my plants to create a narrative, a story—I'm a storyteller. I create a sense of place and history, a contrast and conversation between objects, to ignite other people's imaginations. After knowing and writing that story, I want to ask people, "What does that do for you, and what is the subconscious effect on your day from that?" Setting up different areas in my home does that for me automatically. I feel their effects on me, and they ignite my creativity and sense of place.

Your work is so colorful—do you have a favorite hue on the color wheel?

The turquoise/blue-green family. To cool me down. It makes me feel peaceful.

I love the way colors interact with one another. Being biracial (half Jewish and half African American), I rely on pieces that rely on contrast to be what they want to be. Being half and half is like being yin and yang. Part of why I am successful is that I have a duality inside me from two different cultures. I love the beauty of that contrast and what it brings. I try to explore that in my design work, create wild contrasts that people normally wouldn't put together and see all the beauty that it creates.

If you were a crystal, which crystal would you be?

Iron Pyrite, because its multifaceted nature speaks to me. I love how it stands out. It has a powerful feeling about it in the way it interacts with the other crystals because it is so highly reflective. I relate to that because I have a lot of different authentic faces that I show to people.

SACRED GEOMETRY: THE POWER OF CRYSTAL GRIDDING

Every crystal possesses a unique energy that affects everything in its surroundings. By creating a crystal grid, you can increase that sphere of influence by combining the energies of various types of crystals so that they work together. It's like a whole team of healers focusing on one specialized area. Strength in numbers, right?

WHAT IS A CRYSTAL GRID, EXACTLY?

Crystal grids are made by placing stones in a geometric pattern with the specific purpose of directing energy toward a goal. The stones or crystals are then charged by your intention and energy. Crystal grids can be used for goals that are large or small, vague or specific, like calling new energy into your life, or getting a raise within the next two months at work. By combining your intentions with the power of crystals, and the power of Sacred Geometry (which we'll get into a bit later), you can create a visual narrative and a tool for manifesting your thoughts so that they become reality. The crystals on your grid should always be placed with intention, never randomly. Crystal grids are designed with many components, and each part has a specific purpose.

CRYSTAL GRIDDING HOW-TO

What You'll Need

- A sheet of paper with your intentions, goals, and manifestations written on it
- Master Stone or Focus Stone—your center crystal
- Way Stones

- Desire Stones
- Barrier and Dispeller Stones
- A Clear Quartz crystal point for activation
- A cloth or a photo to be used as a backdrop
- Accent items like candles or talismans

Instructions

1. *Find a peaceful spot:* This should be a safe location for your grid where it won't be disturbed.

2. *Cleanse your space:* Burn sage, palo santo, or other sacred herbs, just as you would when cleansing a room of unwanted energy or when building an altar (see page 158). Add candles, incense, flowers, or music to set the scene, if you like.

3. *Set an intention for your grid:* Your intention is what juices up the crystals. Take a few deep breaths, then write your intention on a sheet of paper. Fold this sheet of paper and place it in the center of your crystal grid.

4. *Choose a pattern:* This is where Sacred Geometry, a system that assigns sacred meanings to certain geometric shapes, comes in. The Sacred Geometry pattern you choose for your grid should align with your grid's intention. Pattern options include: Ashok Chakra, Borromean Rings, Circles, Eye of Horus, Hexagons, Five Platonic Solids, Flower of Life, Mandelas, Metatron's Cube, Pentagons, Pyramids, Seeds of Life, Squares, Spirals, Toroids, Triangles, and Vesica Pisces. Google these patterns, along with "Sacred Geometry," to learn more about their particular shapes and their meanings. You can find Sacred Geometry patterns online to print out, buy crystal gridding cloths with shapes printed on them, or just go freehand.

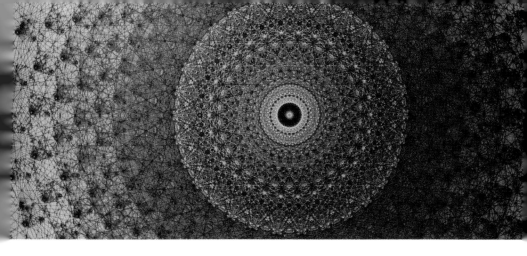

5. *Add sparkle:* Choose crystals and stones that are aligned with your intention and that will visually and energetically enhance your grid. For example, if you are looking to create an abundance grid, choose stones associated with wealth like Green Aventurine, Citrine, Jade, and Iron Pyrite. If you are creating a wellness grid, use blue and purple healing stones like Amethyst, Aquamarine, Fluorite, and Turquoise.

6. *Place your Focus/Master Stone:* Located in the center of your crystal grid, the Master Stone's primary purpose is to collect energy, amplify it, and channel it through the rest of the grid. There are two schools of thought on when to place the Master Stone: It should be either the very first or the very last crystal added on the grid. I like to place the Master Stone first, and I think of it as starting on the inside and working outward, energetically and physically speaking.

7. *Choose your path:* The path on your crystal grid is the line of energy that flows through the grid from the Master Stone at the center to the Way Stones (which further amplify your grid's energy) to the Desire Stones (which represent the ultimate outcome of your grid). Your path (determined by the grid design you choose) draws on Sacred Geometry teachings and principles

to align, transmit, and guide our energy to achieve our goals. The path is vital because it establishes which way energy flows through the grid. Once you've established your path, you are ready to place your crystals onto your chosen Sacred Geometry layout.

8. *Place your Way Stones:* Your Master Stone sends energy to your Way Stones, which further amplify your grid's energy. Way Stones are "stepping stones" that represent the various points on your journey toward the intention you have set for your grid. Way Stones help you take things one step at a time, while focusing on the bigger picture.

9. *Place your Desire Stones:* Your Desire Stones represent the ultimate outcome of your grid. Energy flows through the Way Stones into the Desire Stones, dispersing energy that will allow you to achieve that outcome.

10. *Add a Protection Circle:* Creating a Protection Circle around the perimeter of your grid keeps away any unwanted energy, and provides a designated space for focusing and amplifying your intentions. Adding a Protection Circle is like carrying an umbrella when the forecast is looking unpredictable: You may not need it, but why risk outside influences interfering with your work and energy? Barrier and Dispeller Stones are used here in equal numbers and are alternated for even coverage.

11. *Activate your grid:* Once you have arranged all your stones, say a prayer and visualize the intention for your grid having been achieved. Next take your Clear Quartz crystal point and, starting from the perimeter of your grid, trace a path from one stone to the next to connect them all energetically (like "connecting the dots" when you were a kid). Congratulations! Your crystal grid is officially activated and finished. You can now add candles, talismans, and other energy-healing tools around the outskirts of your grid.

12. *Grid life:* It's important that you engage with the energy of your grid regularly, just as you would with an altar. Gaze at the stones,

read the written intention you've placed on your grid, and visualize the outcome on a daily basis.

13. *Post-grid:* Once assembled, I like to leave a crystal grid intact for at least an entire moon cycle. Since we call new energy in on the new moon, I'll create a grid on a new moon, then dismantle it on a full moon, when we traditionally release energy into the universe. However, you can start and finish on any day of the month that resonates with you. Dismantle your grid by taking it apart in the order in which it was put together. Be sure to cleanse the stones before using them again, and finish by burning sage or palo santo to clear the energy of your space.

Common Crystals to Use in Gridding:

- **WHEN YOUR INTENTION IS ABUNDANCE:** Citrine, Green Aventurine, Amber, Jade, Iron Pyrite
- **WHEN YOUR INTENTION IS LOVE:** Rose Quartz, Emerald, Ruby Fuchsite, Morganite, Rhodonite
- **WHEN YOUR INTENTION IS SERENITY:** Amethyst, Howlite, Moonstone, Ocean Jasper
- **WHEN YOUR INTENTION IS TRUTH/COMMUNICATION:** Blue Kyanite, Lapis Lazuli, Sodalite, Blue Onyx

DIY: THE SUNBURST GRID

The Sunburst Grid is one of the most common and popular crystal grid formations, and it's a great one to start with. Here are basic instructions for assembling one:

1. *Begin by finding a peaceful spot* and cleansing your space before you begin, as described on page 170.

2. ***Set your intention:*** Let's imagine we want to radiate success in business out into the world. We want to call in "being-seen" and making more money.

3. ***Place your Focus/Master Stone (Center Position):*** Use Citrine here, as it is the "Stone of Business" and helps call in monetary abundance. Yellow is also a color that relates to our 3rd/Solar Plexus Chakra, which is our personal power center.

4. ***Place your Way Stones (Middle Position):*** Use single-terminated Green Aventurine points for luck and money.

5. ***Place your Desire Stones (Outer Position):*** Use single-terminated Clear Quartz points here for clarity, vision, and amplification. Notice in the illustration how the energy of these stones is radiating outward into the universe.

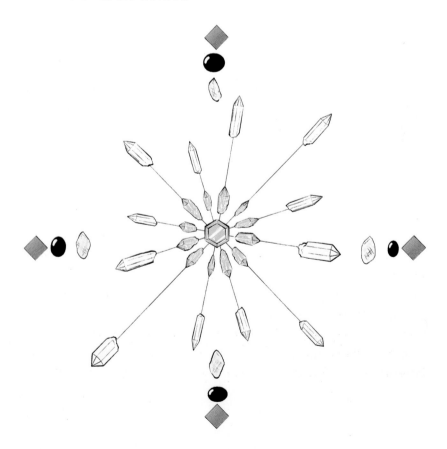

6. ***Place your Perimeter Stones (your Protection Circle):*** These outer stones should support your desired outcome and protect the perimeter of the grid. I chose Iron Pyrite, Black Obsidian, and Herkimer Diamonds. Iron Pyrite carries a strong manifesting vibration; it represents the earth and grounding, and carries masculine energy. (When we want to put something out into the world, we need to engage with the Divine Masculine side that lives within each of us. This energy helps us get it done by moving from point A to point B, gives us the drive to plan and execute work projects, encourages goal-driven thoughts and actions, etc.) Black Obsidian is grounding and protecting. Herkimer Diamond is added for additional radiance.

7. Follow steps 11 to 13 on pages 172–73 for crystal grid magic!

WHAT ELSE CAN I DO WITH CRYSTALS?

This is one of the most common questions I get from my clients. And the answer is, everything and anything! There are so many fascinating modern uses for crystals. In this section I want to share them with you, and I'm going to introduce you to some of the creatives out there who are doing game-changing work with crystals in their respective fields.

GEM ELIXIRS

Did you know you can drink your crystals, too? A gem elixir, also known as "crystal essence" or "crystal water," is drinking water infused with the positive energy of crystals. Gems have been used to energetically charge water since the times of ancient Greece. When water is infused with gems, the energy of the gemstones purifies the water and can "program" it to do certain things, like boost concentration and energy, increase self-confidence, alleviate pain, temper allergies, and even improve conditions in your love life. When you drink a gem elixir, your body absorbs the energy of the crystal or crystals used to make it. Gem elixirs are an easy and convenient way to work with the vibrational energies of crystals. They're very easy to make, even if you're a beginner, and they can be stored for later use.

There are two ways to make gem elixirs: the "direct" method and the "indirect" method. The direct method involves soaking your crystals directly in water, but this can be potentially dangerous if your stones contain toxic elements. I do not recommend the direct method unless you are 100 percent sure that your crystals are nontoxic and nonporous, and you have consulted a professional first. Instead, I strongly recommend the indirect method, which is safest for beginners and for all crystal types, because the elixir waters don't come into direct contact with your crystals. When I create gem elixirs, I also like to use multiple types of stones and crystals to create a synergy blend, which is useful for bringing together the vibrations of several stones.

DIY GEM WATER

Gem water is easy to make at home, but keep in mind that it should be prepared for immediate use, unless you add a preservative to it. You can store it in an airtight container in the refrigerator, but not for longer than 2 to 3 days.

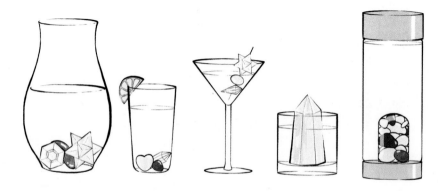

Tools

- The crystals you plan to use, including Clear Quartz as an energy amplifier
- Two clean glass containers, one large and one smaller (The exact size of the containers doesn't matter, but the smaller container must be able to fit inside the larger one with some wiggle room between them.)
- Two clean, dark-colored glass bottles, one large and one small with a dropper top
- Springwater, rainwater, or distilled water
- 80-proof or higher vodka (If you are alcohol-free, you can substitute any variety of vinegar. The vodka or vinegar acts as a preservative for your gem water.)

Directions

1. Cleanse and charge the crystals you plan to use, then lay out your tools in a clean, dry space. Approach this process with a calm, positive, refreshed state of mind. Don't mix elixirs after a challenging day at work, or when you are feeling sick.
2. Get centered and grounded, and take some deep breaths. State an intention for your elixir, silently or out loud. As an example, you can make a "Love" elixir using Rose Quartz and Clear Quartz, and your intention for this elixir could be, "I ask to call healthy and loving relationships into my life." Or if you are making an elixir that will help you quit smoking using Amethyst, your intention could be something like, "I do not allow my addictions to rule my life."
3. Place your crystals in the smaller glass container, and place that container inside the larger glass container. Carefully fill the larger

container with water, being mindful not to get any water into the smaller container.

4. Cover or seal the containers. Set them in a place, either in sunlight, moonlight, or in a sacred space, where they won't be disturbed for at least 6 hours.

5. Remove the inner container of crystals and carefully pour the "charged" water from the larger outer container (this charged water is also referred to as the "mother elixir" or "essence") into the larger of the two glass bottles. Fill the bottle halfway with your essence, and fill the rest of the bottle with vodka or vinegar. Seal the bottle tightly.

6. Fill the smaller glass bottle with the remaining essence. You can use springwater or distilled water to dilute the essence, or you may want to leave it at its full concentration. Seal the bottle. Keep the larger bottle in the fridge; since it contains a preservative, you can store it for a longer period of time. The smaller bottle is for immediate use and is easier to use because it has a dropper lid for easy use, is easy to travel with, etc. Either apply 4–8 drops directly to the tongue with dropper or 4–8 drops to an 8oz. glass of water and stir.

7. Clean your tools and store them for future use. You can simply pour any unused essence into the sink, or you can ceremoniously pour it out onto the earth while expressing your gratitude for the process.

KITCHEN MAGIC!

There are hundreds of gem water recipes out there, so I turned to one of my top experts, LA-based Chinese medicine doctor Mona Dinari, for a great DIY recipe you can easily make at home. This recipe is ideal for treating jet lag and EMF exposure. Thanks, Dr. Mona!

You will need the following tumbled crystals (meaning they have been smoothed and polished in a crystal tumbler):

- Green Tourmaline
- Rhodonite
- Amethyst

Directions

1. Cleanse your stones by soaking them overnight, but not more than eight hours, in a glass container using sparkling mineral water. Cover the container top with a napkin or cloth.
2. Pour out the soaking water and replace with 8 ounces of still spring water overnight or longer, keeping the container out of the sun.
3. Now the elixir us ready. Drink 2 ounces of it twice a day.
4. At the end of the day, add 4 ounces of water to the original glass with the stones and leave it overnight. This way, you always maintain the original concentration.

Preferred types of mineral water to wash the stones are naturally sparkling waters such as Gerolsteiner and Apollinaris, any type of springwater, or filtered water.

Types of springwater to make the elixir (please purchase in a glass bottle)

- Mountain valley spring water
- Oregon water
- Eternal
- Glacier water

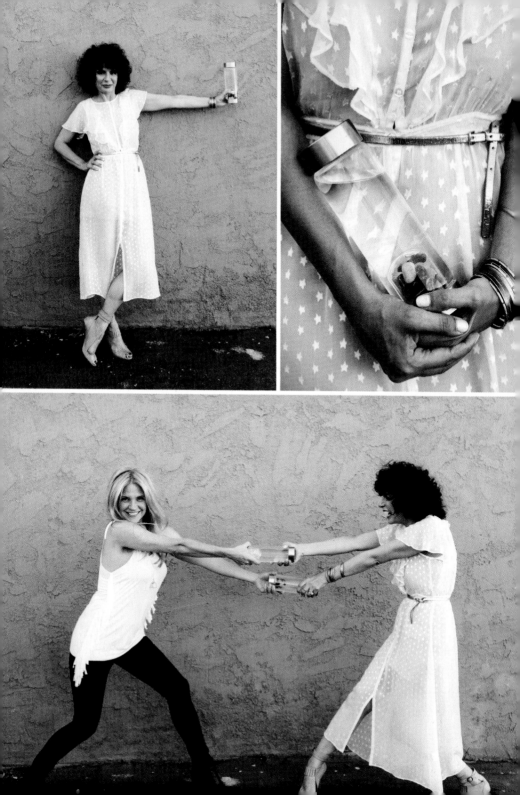

Interview with Anjanette Sinesio, Founder of Gem-Water

ANJANETTE IS THE OWNER OF GEM-WATER, a company that sells beautifully designed water bottles that you can use to infuse your drinking water with the healing power of stones. We originally met at a press event in New York City, and we've since become close friends, bonding over the fact that my past life was in fashion, and hers began in the high-end-jewelry industry.

When did you first get into crystals?

My fascination with crystals began was when I was about eight years old, visiting my dad in San Francisco. My parents were divorced, and most of the year I lived with my mom in New Jersey. I wanted to bring a gift back for my mom, and we went shopping and I saw this gorgeous Amethyst geode. I knew that was what I had to get her, and it's my earliest memory of being really drawn to the energy and beauty of crystals.

How did Gem-Water start?

I started Gem-Water after coming across a German company, VitaJuwel, that was making gem water. I contacted VitaJuwel founder

Ewald Eisen, and Gem-Water was born in 2016. As a jewelry designer and gem lover, I had this realization that for twenty-plus years, I'd been helping women adorn themselves on the outside with jewelry and gems. Now I had this opportunity to help them harness the power of gems to create beauty on the inside. This insight was incredibly powerful to me, and I knew that this was now part of my calling.

What's up with the little pod of crystals in the center of the water bottle?

So many people ask this question—"How does the pod work if the stones aren't 'touching' the water?" Many people put their stones right into the water, but this "direct" method is only right for certain stones. Others can release toxins into your water. The pod encases the stones, which is the safest method, and their vibration still affects the water—the glass doesn't prevent the transfer of energy. All you have to do is wait 7 to 10 minutes for the crystals to work their magic!

What is Gem-Water's number one seller?

Our Wellness Gem-Water Bottle, which contains Amethyst, Rose Quartz, and Clear Quartz, is our top-selling product, I think because the colors of the stones are so beautiful, and because women's wellness is such a hot topic right now. People are really beginning to understand the role gemstones can play in their well-being.

What other Gem-Water products are there, in addition to the water bottles?

In addition to our Gem-Water bottles that you can take on the go, our product line includes gem vials/wands that you can put into our Era Decanter to serve gem water from the table at home. We also have our little Gemstone Droplet, which is a single-serving gemstone vial that you can put in a glass of water, or in a glass of red wine! We also have a Vino Vial and Vino Decanter for infusing a full bottle of wine with Amethyst. Believe it or not, the practice of enhancing wine with Amethyst goes back to the ancient Greeks!

DO NOT DRINK THESE!

It's important to do your research before you make gem water at home. As I've mentioned, certain crystals can release toxins when immersed in water, and shouldn't be used for direct-method gem water at all. Crystals that you never, ever want to drink include those containing asbestos, copper, lead, mercury, or sulfur; shiny, metallic stones that can rust when placed in water for prolonged periods; salt-based crystals, like Selenite, because they dissolve; and blue and green stones, especially brightly colored ones, as they contain copper and/or arsenic. Here is a list of the stones that should NOT be used for gem water:

- Amazonite (contains copper)
- Aquamarine (contains aluminum)
- Azurite (contains copper)
- Black Tourmaline (contains aluminum)
- Cavansite (contains copper)
- Celestite (contains strontium)
- Peacock Ore (contains copper and sulfur and can rust)
- Charoite
- Chrysocolla (contains copper)
- Cinnabar (contains mercury)
- Emerald (contains aluminum)
- Fluorite (contains fluorine)
- Garnet (contains aluminum)
- Galena (contains lead)
- Hematite (will rust, but not toxic)
- Iolite (contains aluminum)
- Kunzite (contains aluminum)
- Labradorite (contains aluminum)
- Lapis Lazuli (contains pyrite)
- Lepidolite (contains aluminum and mica)
- Magnetite (will rust, but not toxic)
- Malachite (contains copper)
- Moldavite (contains aluminum oxide)
- Moonstone (contains aluminum)
- Morganite (contains aluminum)
- Prehnite (contains aluminum)
- Pyrite (contains sulfur)
- Realgar (contains arsenic)
- Ruby (contains aluminum)
- Sapphire (contains aluminum)
- Selenite (friable, meaning tiny shards may break off in water, but not toxic)
- Serpentine (may contain asbestos)
- Shaman Quartz (contains sulfur, pyrite, and marcasite)
- Sodalite (contains aluminum)
- Spinel (contains aluminum)
- Stilbite (contains aluminum)
- Sugilite (contains aluminum)
- Sulfur Quartz (contains sulfur)
- Sunstone (contains aluminum)
- Tanzanite (contains aluminum)
- Tiger's Eye (contains asbestos)
- Topaz (contains aluminum)
- Tourmaline (contains aluminum)
- Turquoise (contains copper and aluminum)

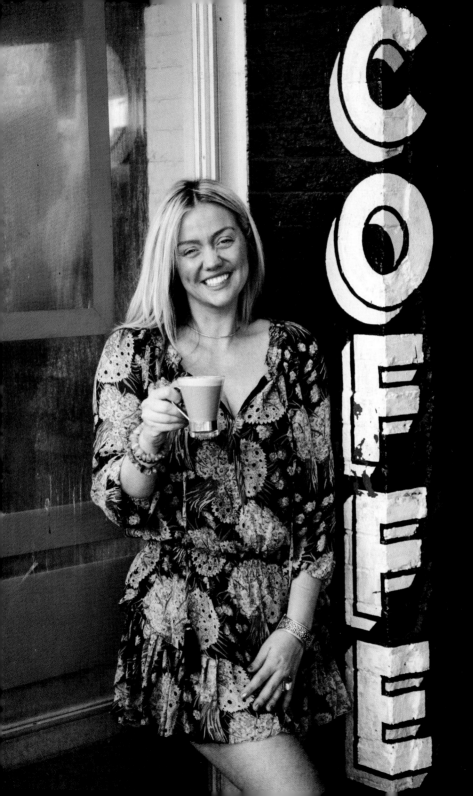

ANOTHER WAY TO DRINK YOUR CRYSTALS: THE AMETHYST-DUSTED GEODE LATTE

My friend and fellow Virgo Madeleine Murphy is the creator of the purple Amethyst-Dusted Geode Latte, a beautiful and delicious way to get your daily crystal fix. Madi co-owns The End Brooklyn café in Williamsburg, home of the Geode Latte, as well as Montauk Juice Factory out east. Her Williamsburg shop sells delicious hot plant-based drinks and juices, along with jewelry, skincare products, and other crystal trinkets any magical mer-babe may need in her daily life. In case you can't make it out to Williamsburg anytime soon, Madi has been kind enough to share the recipe for her signature sparkly brew, so that you can be the beverage "it" girl at your next Moon Circle!

The purple Amethyst-Dusted Geode Latte is an excellent way to bring the healing powers of amethyst into your life. The latte, infused with an Amethyst elixir, stimulates the Third Eye and Crown Chakras and enhances cognitive perception, while heightening your imagination and intuition, and strengthening your emotional field. And the luscious purple-hued superfoods it contains, maqui berry and hibiscus, have antioxidant, anti-inflammatory, anticarcinogenic, and healing effects.

Madi, if you were a crystal, which one would you be?

A mix of Aqua Aura Quartz—because I am like a blue, shiny, iridescent mermaid—and Smoky Quartz, to match my brooding, internal, thinking, witchy side.

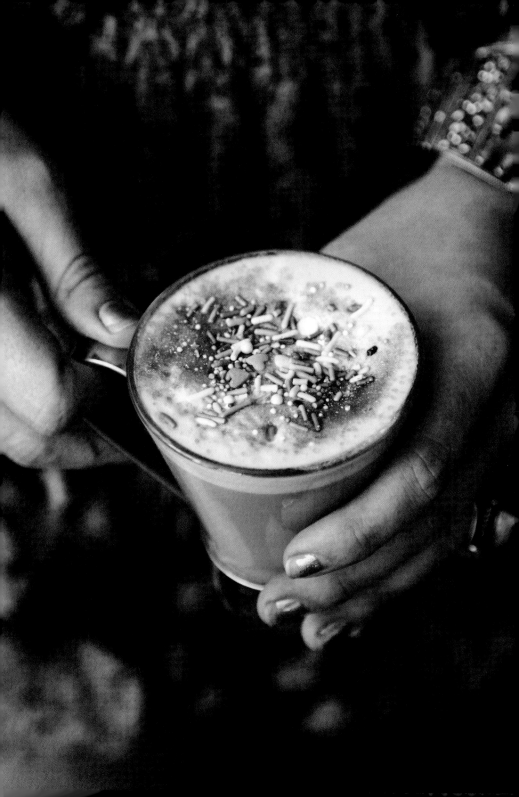

The End Brooklyn's
Amethyst-Dusted Geode Latte

Makes 2

1 or 2 medium-size tumbled
  Amethyst stones, cleansed
2 cups hibiscus or mulberry tea
1 cup oat milk (or nondairy milk of
  your choice)
1 tablespoon maqui berry powder,
  plus more for garnish
1 tablespoon coconut oil

1 tablespoon maca powder
1 tablespoon liquid crystal silica
2 teaspoons tocos rice bran powder
1 teaspoon locally harvested honey
  (Manuka, if you feel like splurging)
3 drops of colloidal silver
Dried lavender buds, for garnish

1. At least 72 hours in advance, follow the instructions on page 179 using the Amethysts to make an Amethyst gem elixir.* (You'll need at least 2 cups elixir for this recipe.)
2. Put the hibiscus or mulberry tea in a large glass measuring cup or heat-safe pitcher. Bring 2 cups of the Amethyst gem elixir to a boil in a small saucepan and pour it over the tea. Steep the tea until it has a rich, jewel-tone hue to get all the crystal-y goodness in there. Discard hibiscus or mulberry tea leaves when done.
3. Add the oat milk to the tea and stir to combine. Add the maqui, coconut oil, maca, silica, tocos, honey, and colloidal silver.
4. To mix the ingredients and simultaneously add a nice froth, use a handheld milk frother. Place the frother right in the glass for 15 to 30 seconds, or more, as desired, to up the cozy vibes. Alternatively, pour the tea mixture into a saucepan and whisk vigorously over low heat for 60 to 90 seconds.
5. Garnish with some maqui berry powder and dried lavender buds.

As amazing as it looks, this latte is also one of the healthiest, most loving things you can do for your body. Enjoy!

For extra crystalline magic, you can also infuse your Amethyst elixir with polished Rose Quartz or Citrine.

CRYSTALS IN RITUAL BATHING

Ritual bathing has long been practiced for hygiene, health, relaxation and for spiritual purposes. Bathing emporiums started popping up as early as the third century, and they became *the* fashionable places to be seen and get clean. Patrons would socialize, conduct business deals, eat, and rejuvenate while bathing. What's the modern-day recipe for purity, hygiene, and ritual purification? I recommend incorporating crystals into your bathing routine! Saltwater baths are an easy way to get your aura squeaky clean and free of unwanted energy.

HOW DOES SALT WATER HELP?

- Saltwater baths can help to relieve muscle aches and pains, and increase circulation.
- Your body needs the essential trace minerals found in bath salts.
- The skin is an organ of elimination, and saltwater soaking will draw toxins and heavy metals from the tissues.
- Salt water draws bacteria from the skin, so it can help with skin ailments, in addition to increasing your overall dewy glow.

    P.S. *Take a saltwater bath no more than once a week. Since this is an energy exchange between you, the water, and the crystals, once or twice a month is ideal.*

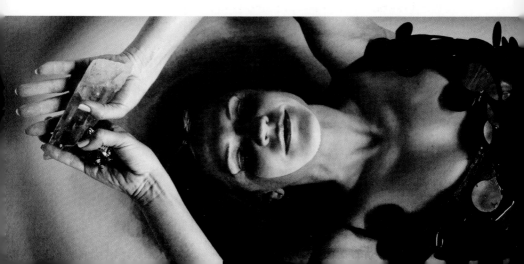

BATH TIME! SYNC IT UP WITH THE MOON

What You'll Need

- Bath salts (unrefined sea salt, pink Himalayan salt, or Epsom salts)
- Your favorite energizing and purifying crystals
- Candles, incense, herbs, flowers, scented oils

Instructions

1. First and foremost, remember that this is YOU time. Place the "Do Not Disturb" sign on your bathroom door, and put your phone on airplane mode. Create an experience that appeals to all your senses: Light candles or incense; add herbs, flowers, and oils to the water; and don't forget a relaxing playlist.

2. Make crystal bathing a regular self-care ritual by deciding on a lunar phase to work with: New moons are best for manifesting and calling in new things, while full moons are best for releasing unwanted energy and releasing what is no longer serving you.

3. Make sure that your tub is clean, and take a quick shower before indulging in your ritual bath.

4. Fill your bathtub with warm to hot water. Temperature is a personal preference.

5. Crystalize your bathwater by adding several generous handfuls of salt. Use unrefined sea salt, pink Himalayan salt, or Epsom salts. DO NOT use regular table salt, as this has added anticaking agents and has been put through a refinement process that removes the minerals that cleanse, purify, and rejuvenate our bodies.

6. Drop your favorite (nonporous) crystals into the water. The same crystals that should not be used in gem water should also be avoided for crystal bathing. As a beginner, the best bath stones to start with are Rose Quartz, Amethyst, or Clear Quartz. If you

want to call in love, place a few pieces of cleansed and tumbled Rose Quartz in the bath with you. If you want increased stamina and focus, work with polished or tumbled Clear Quartz. Refer to the go-to crystal lists in chapters 2 and 4 for other intentions that you are trying to achieve with your ritual bathing. You can hold your crystals while bathing, place them on your body, or submerge them in the water.

7. Soak for 30 minutes or so. While in the tub, set an intention to call in or release energies.

8. Try to air-dry when you get out of the bath. If possible, don't take another shower or bath for 24 hours.

9. Time to drain the tub. Offer a little thank you to the universe for the much-needed "me time" and pull the plug with respect, gratitude, and intention.

10. Extra credit! Before draining the tub, collect some of your bathwater in a drinking glass or other glass container. Energetically and physically, this water now carries your energy and literally your DNA. As an offering of thanks to the earth for the water, pour the water at the base of a tree, in a garden, or in a grassy area.

CRYSTALS FOR YOUR CLOSET!

Let's explore one of the most sacred spaces in the home: your closet. Your wardrobe says so much about who you are and the energy you put out into the world. So it's important that the good vibes begin in your closet itself. The Style Rituals Closet Cleanse, where I add crystals to my clients' closets, is one of my signature services. Here are my favorite Closet Cleanse tips and tricks:

• Incorporate fêng shui principles and directionally grid the four corners of your closet with crystals, just like you would the individual rooms in your home.

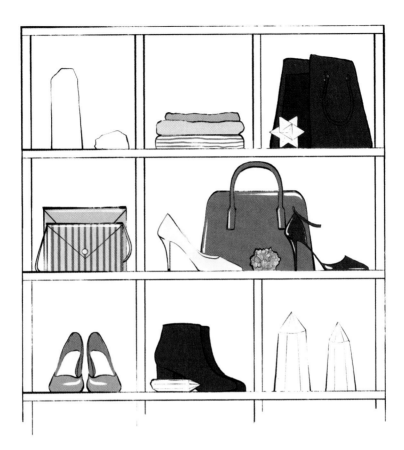

- Set up a crystal grid within the closet (see the section on crystal gridding on page 169).
- Selenite, the "cosmic cleaning lady," is a must-have in your closet. Selenite keeps everything in your closet energetically fresh— it's like energetic moth balls (without the smell)! Selenite can go in the four corners of your closet where dense energy tends to accumulate like dust bunnies. It's also great in closed places like drawers and shoe boxes.
- Match crystals with the energy you want to infuse into certain types of clothing. Place Citrine near work ensembles, Bloodstone near fitness gear, and Rose Quartz near lingerie.

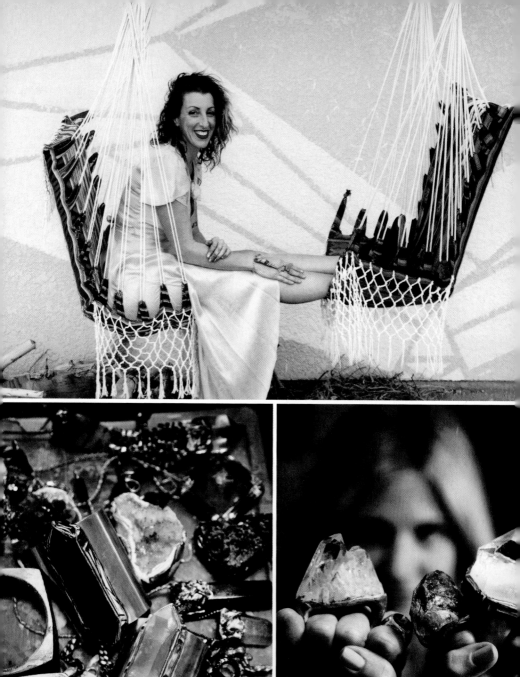
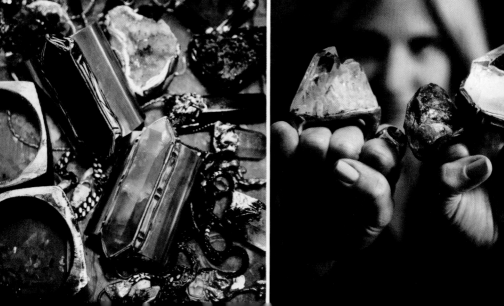

Interview with Adina Mills, Crystal Jeweler to the Stars

I FIRST MET ADINA while adventuring in Joshua Tree, where she was having a sample sale at her studio. I'm not the only one who hearts Adina's larger-than-life "wearable altar" statement pieces: You can find her designs around the necks and fingers of celebs like Erykah Badu, Lena Dunham, Pink, and Bjork, and in an Anthropologie near you.

When did you get into crystals?

When I was a child. I was always hiking with family to tide pools and collecting beautiful rocks, shells, crystals, and anything nature-related!

When did you start your jewelry business?

Fifteen years ago, I began making jewelry. I made pieces for myself, and then for my sister, who has a massive crystals collection, and for my friends. I was just doing it as a creative outlet and hadn't thought about starting a business, but then I started seeing people's reactions to my pieces, and things just sort of snowballed from there. I began selling my jewelry at art fairs and festivals around LA, and I eventually road tripped in a motorhome across the country to New York City, which is where my business really took off. I met the buyer for Shopbop, who decided to carry my line, and that opened a lot of doors. Today I sell in boutiques globally, and I don't follow seasons. Each piece I create is one of a kind, since I am working with Mother Nature.

If you were a crystal, which crystal would you be?

Clear Quartz. I LOVE quartz, because it amplifies every possible emotion.

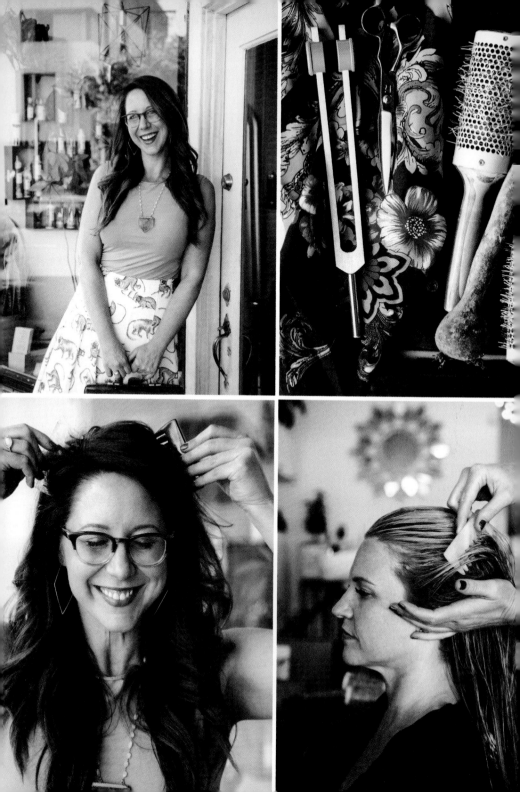

Interview with Andi Scarbrough, the Crystal Hair Revivalist

MY DEAR FRIEND AND TRUSTED HAIRDRESSER ANDI is the creator of CrownWorks Crystal Combs and hair treatments, which are celebrated by her private clients as well as celebrities, beauty experts, and beauty editors. Andi, a former L'Oréal teaching facilitator, has been doing cut and color for fifteen years. She's the owner of Framed Salon in LA, a Reiki practitioner, and a healer with a degree in spiritual psychology from the University of Santa Monica.

When did your love of crystals begin?

When I was a little girl in Texas, I would wander along the lake edge and pick up stones. I got my first rock tumbler at age nine, and I still have many of the stones I collected back them. Now that I live in California, I'm surrounded by boulders and mountains, and they are a constant source of inspiration for me.

How did you start CrownWorks hair treatments?

Early on in my career as a hairdresser, I was already deep into crystals, searching for stones that would aid with issues I was struggling with, like restless sleep, nightmares, clarity of thought, and patience. The first crystals I gravitated toward were Rose Quartz, Fluorite, Selenite, and Watermelon Tourmaline. By the time I started CrownWorks, my hairstyling station at work already looked like a rock shop, as did the stations of all the other stylists in my salon! So I started using the stones as a point of resonance in my beauty work. Clients would sit down in my chair, and I would give them a stone to hold while I cut and colored their hair, and I could see their energy shift.

Can you talk a bit about CrownWorks Crystal Combs?

A year and a half ago I had a dream about running a comb made of crystals through a client's hair, so I decided to make it reality and started searching for a source. My combs are hand-cut and German-engineered, and I sell them in Amethyst, Rose Quartz, Snow Quartz, Black Obsidian, Labradorite, and Carnelian. When you run a crystal comb through your hair, you are using the power of gemstone energy to influence your entire energetic system, including improving your circulation and stimulating blood flow to the scalp.

CRYSTALS IN THE HEALTH AND BEAUTY WORLD

Wash, comb, spray, nip, prick, tuck, poke, roll, rinse, and lather up! Words every girl is used to hearing when reading a glossy, but did you know all these terms apply to working with gems, too? Crystals can strengthen skin's elasticity, fight free radicals, and combat wrinkles, plus give new life to your hair, pump up your chi, *and* keep your "down there" in shape.

Interview with Rachel Lang and Heidi Frederick, Cofounders of FaceLove

I MET RACHEL AND HEIDI at the inaugural #InGoopHealth event in Los Angeles in 2017. I was beckoned to come sit in a striped deck chair turned facial throne covered with sheepskins and given a sidecar of Pamplemousse LaCroix. Team FaceLove's modern beauty wellness ritual consists of ancient massage techniques, acupressure, hands-on healing, and a chilled Jade Crystal roller to complete the self-proclaimed "facial choreography" session. The dynamic duo claims their techniques boost circulation and will make you feel more centered (and personally, my client feedback after our session together was that I felt like I had just had sex. Yeah, it was *that* good!). If that isn't an endorsement to book a session immediately, then I don't know what is!

How did you two meet?

RACHEL: Heidi and I met on the playground in New York City as new moms. We instantly became best friends, and then we became business partners in a hot New York minute because we shared so many of the same practices and principles within our respective crafts. Heidi was a massage therapist, working with ballet dancers and musicians, inspired to go into her craft by her Japanese stepmother, and I was working as a facialist and global educator with the Aveda Institute.

When did you start FaceLove?

RACHEL: Three years ago I wrote the idea on a bar napkin. I was born with a cleft lip and have had several facial surgeries, and I've been doing facials for twenty-five years. When I was working as a facialist and global educator at Aveda, I invented the "Non-Product Facial," also called a "Water Facial," for clients who didn't want products on their face or messing up their hair. I started studying massage techniques from around the world and developed what I call "FaceLove choreography," which is based on the idea that the muscles in your face are all connected to your emotions. Holding an expression like "resting bitch face" can actually create muscle atrophy, sagging, and face posture changes. But my techniques tone the facial muscles and create metabolic transformation within the skin and tissue. It's preventative medicine.

When did you start using the Jade roller in your treatments?

RACHEL: My mom inspired this treatment. She used to do ice cube massages to tighten her face, so I began wondering what an iced jade roller would do. I really loved using a paintbrush and Black Tourmaline gems to create an energetic massage. Then one day I walked into the well-known SoHo store Pearl River Mart and I discovered the Jade roller, which blends gems and painting! I decided then and there that I had to understand this ancient tool and incorporate it into our treatments. We start our Jade roller treatment with warm heat from a sauna, and then we use the roller to increase blood flow. We use Jade because it's not only a coveted and celebrated stone in Asia, but also because it's soothing and cooling, and has infrared healing properties and helps to promote homeostasis.

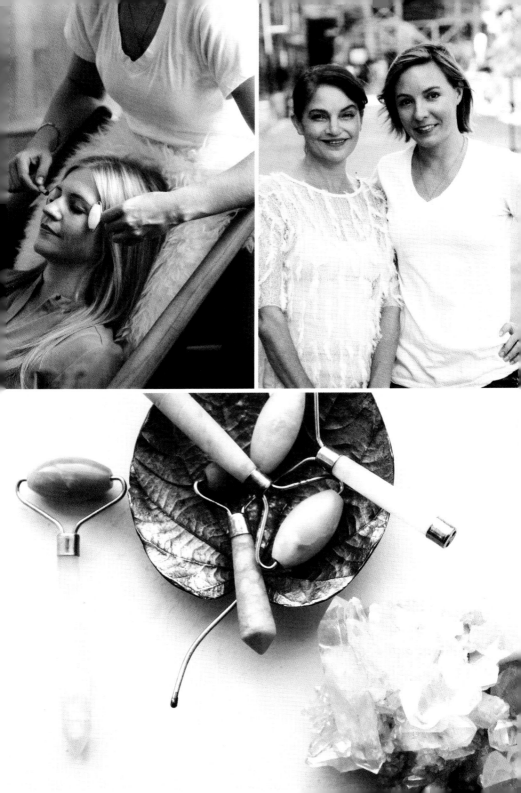

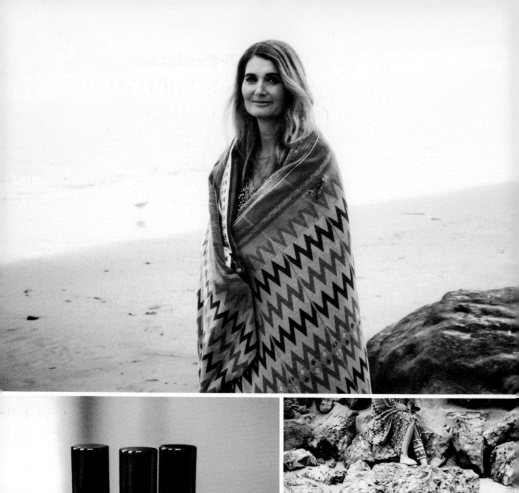

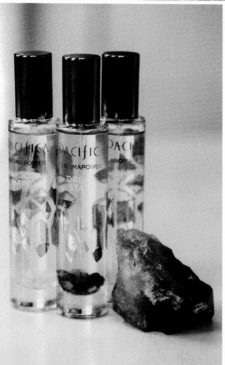

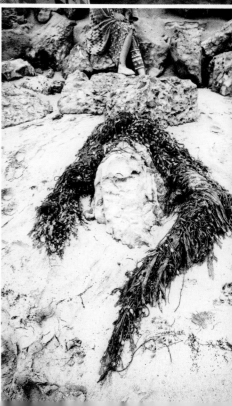

Interview with Brook Harvey-Taylor, Founder of Pacifica Beauty

BROOK HARVEY-TAYLOR IS THE FOUNDER and creative director of Pacifica Beauty, a 100 percent vegan natural makeup, skincare, and fragrance company. After meeting Brook, I officially designated her "High Priestess of the Olfactory." The cherry on top? Many of her thoughtfully curated, beautifully designed products are made with gemstones!

When did you get into crystals?

I have been into stones, rocks, and crystals since I was little. I grew up on a cattle ranch in Montana, and I would ride my horse around our land, pick herbs, find stones, and play "medicine woman." My mom was a hippie, earth mother–type. She was diagnosed with breast cancer and became really conscious of what she put on her skin or ingested. She was an early adopter and proponent of natural products. During college, I worked at a health food store, where I got to know a healer who used aromatherapy and crystals. I trained with her in essential oils and began making my own perfumes, which I would sell at festivals. This was the beginning of my life as a creative entrepreneur.

What can you tell us about Pacifica?

Perfumes have always been the core of our line; fragrance is in our DNA. Fragrance and perfume connect us to past experiences and possibly even other realms that we can't even comprehend. I can pick up this jasmine scent that smells the same today as it would have in ninth-century Arabia. Fragrance is a powerful vehicle that can take you places. Bringing crystals into our formula was a natural next step. Crystals can change the vibration of water, so I explored how that concept can be applied to oils, scents, and topical products. We don't follow the beauty industry standard of picking skincare according to a person's skin type. I believe in "situational skincare." I want my customers to ask, "Where is my skin today?" Your body is ever-evolving, so why wouldn't your skin's needs change constantly as well?

How do you pick crystals?

I am driven by smell, and everything in my life is grounded by scent. Tuning to the olfactory components of crystals was only natural. When I get into my intuitive space, I decide what type of stone "smells" right with what oil. We launched Pacifica Aromapower roll-on perfumes a year ago; each perfume has an aromatherapeutic benefit and a crystal benefit. This is a space where we integrate stone therapy into perfumes and skin care. More crystal-y products to come!

What stones do you like the smell of best?

All stones have intense and specific odors. One of my favorites is Rose Quartz, as it smells "cold." I also like earth stones—the little pebbles you find while out and about on hikes or in riverbeds.

If you were a crystal, which crystal would you be?

100% an Opal!

Interview with Zoë Taylor-Crane of Paper Crane Apothecary

A WHILE AGO, as I was preparing to do a house clearing and needed a smokeless sage spray alternative as requested by my client, I discovered Zoë's company and her Clean Slate Smoke-Free Smudge Mist. After learning some of the other product names for her gem-infused mists and elixirs, like P.ossible M.urder S.uspect (P.M.S.) and Psychic Vampire Repellant, I knew we would be fast friends and crystal comrades. It turns out I'm not the only one who loves her products—GOOP, *Vogue*, Lea Michele, Alessandra Ambrosio, Debra Messing, and the Hiltons are also big fans.

When did you start Paper Crane Apothecary?

When my son was a year old, I started dabbling with gem elixirs. My son was having a hard time sleeping (which meant we were all having a hard time sleeping), and I created my first gem-infused spray, naming it Dreamcatcher. My libido had also taken a nose dive after having my baby, like many women's, so my first elixir, called Knocking Boots, was meant to remedy that. I shared it with a few friends who immediately said, "Wow, you need to start a business!" I launched my Etsy shop in 2014.

What are your bestsellers, and what's the next product you are releasing?

Our bestselling products are our Clean Slate Smoke-Free Smudge Mist, our Lucky Stars Abundance Mist, and our Psychic Vampire Repellant Protection Mist. We are currently formulating a mist called Mercury Retro Fade Celestial Survival Mist, which will help to ease the dreaded effects of

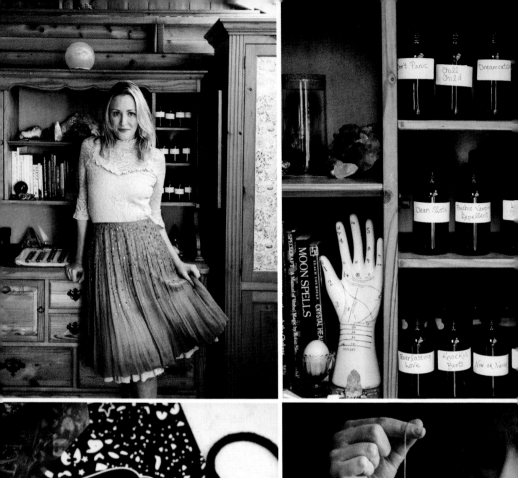

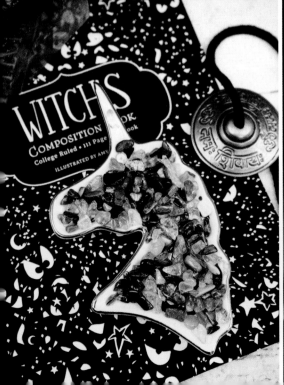

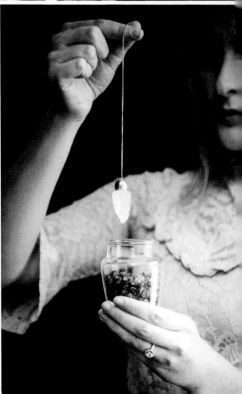

Mercury in retrograde. This blend will be infused with crystals that help with communication (Sodalite and Blue Lace Agate), boost motivation (Carnelian and Tiger's Eye), ease anxiety (Amethyst and Lepidolite), ground and protect the spirit (Black Tourmaline and Smoky Quartz), and help to absorb and reduce the effects of EMFs (Fluorite and Amazonite).

If you were a crystal, which crystal would you be?

Labradorite, because it's mysterious and beautiful when looked at in the right angle, but also has corners of darkness.

CRYSTALS IN HEALTHCARE

East, meet West! Traditional Eastern healing modalities have long used tools like crystals, along with meditation and essential oils, to achieve physical and psychological wellness, and these methods are finally being embraced as complementary and alternative treatments in the West. I'm thrilled to see these traditionally "mystical" remedies reaching a broader audience. Crystals, essential oils, and meditation are being used as healthier, natural substitutes for anxiety meds like Xanax to ease nerves, or to replace pain meds like Lidocaine in certain medical situations. I think that the embracing of these alternative treatments is a sign of our evolution as a culture, and it's an opportunity to open the door to a larger conversation about how these ancient remedies actually work and how we can find more widespread uses for them in the modern world. Spiritual teachings and tools have been kept behind closed doors for too long. They can't help people if we don't have access to them and understand how they work.

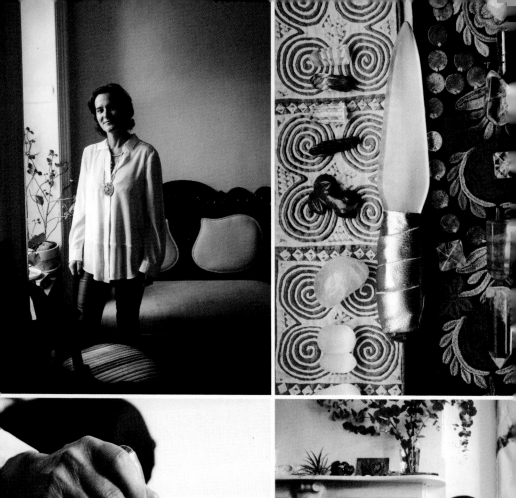
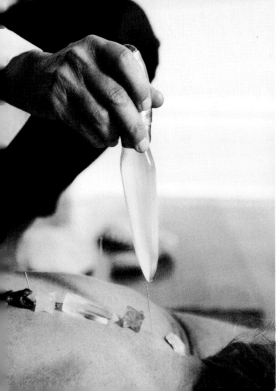
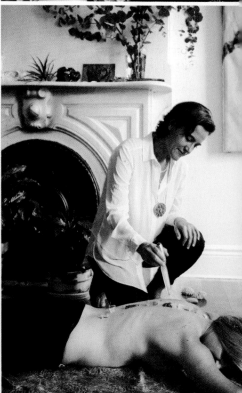

Interview with Consuelo Casarotto, Crystal Acupuncturist

CONSUELO IS MY DEAR FRIEND who also happens to be my go-to New York acupuncturist. We met through a fellow healer who suggested I get to know Consuelo since she incorporated crystals into her acupuncture treatments. Consuelo's bright Manhattan studio is peppered with healing tools from all over the world, including an arsenal of crystal needles.

How did you become an acupuncturist and crystal healer?

I started out as a political science and public policy major, eventually working for the United Nations. After 9/11 I went through a divorce and decided to take a sabbatical year. I spent nine months backpacking through Mexico and Guatemala, where I met shamans and healers, and made my first connection with crystals, finding myself drawn to Jade amulets hand-carved with Mayan mythological figures, Rainbow Obsidian, and Amber. Then I traveled to Italy to be with my aunt who was fighting cancer. I spent day and night by her hospital bed, and I would put crystals all over her room and massage her body with them. She eventually recovered and told me that she'd felt a strong spiritual presence when I was there with her. When I returned to New York, I knew that I needed a new path, and I enrolled in acupuncture school with Master Jeffrey Yuen. That's when my journey as a healer took flight.

How would you describe your practice today?

I am a Licensed Acupuncturist, but "energy healer" would better describe what I do, since I integrate various healing modalities in my work. I run my own practice in Tribeca where I integrate classical and esoteric acupuncture with crystal healing, essential oils therapy, and Sat Nam Rasayan, an ancient healing system introduced by Yogi Bhajan, which uses the contemplative mind to affect change.

What are your favorite crystals to work with in your acupuncture treatments?

I believe that healing is a journey into the deepest reaches of one's heart, and that in order to heal, we must connect with the radiant flame of love, but also with our dark side. This intention is present in all my acupuncture treatments, where I use a combination of crystals that invite connection to both dark and light. My favorite crystals are:

- MOLDAVITE—It invites shifts in consciousness, enabling you to see reality from a renewed perspective.
- TEKTITE—I often place it on the Third Eye or the Throat Chakra to invite communication with higher dimensions.
- AQUAMARINE—I usually place it on the higher Heart Chakra to clarify one's perception, to increase sensitivity and connection to the energy and wisdom of the heart.
- MALACHITE—This is a bridge stone I place between the lower and higher chakras to invite transformation and deep emotional healing.
- OBSIDIAN—A grounding stone, which empowers you to look deep within your darkest shadow, releasing negative conditioning and patterns.
- GREEN TOURMALINE—A mental filter that helps you to see with clarity where you are stuck.
- CLEAR QUARTZ—I always include clear quartz in my healing, as it is the master healer.

If you were a crystal, which one would you be and why?

I would like to be a Black Obsidian. Though my innate nature has me constantly looking up at the stars, I feel drawn to the earthly and grounding powers of Black Obsidian. This stone is like a mirror into the soul, with the power to illuminate that which we are afraid to look at. It invites deep soul healing, and sheds light on one's soul purpose.

Interview with Shiva Rose, Founder of The Local Rose

MY FRIEND SHIVA ROSE is founder of The Local Rose, an LA-based lifestyle brand that celebrates healthy, holistic living. In her breadth of experiences within the health and wellness realm, Shiva became an expert and the modern-day mother of the crystal Yoni Egg. In case you missed it, the Yoni Egg is a stone (Jade, Black Tourmaline, or Rose Quartz) carved into an egg shape and polished to be worn where the sun don't shine. (*Yoni* is another word for "vagina," and you can figure out the rest).

How long have you been working with crystals?

They have been calling to me since I was a little kid. When I was eight I had a cherished set of geodes from a state park that my grandparents gave to me. I'm an Aquarius, so I always wear amethyst. My favorite stones come from the well-known energetic hotspot Mount Shasta, California.

Can you talk to us about the Yoni Egg?

I started using Yoni Eggs five years ago, after learning that Chinese concubines created them thousands of years ago to increase sexual pleasure, awaken sensuality, and promote menstrual health. The Yoni Egg can also be used to strengthen and tone your pelvic floor with special exercises. I tell my clients that this part of the body is like a sacred room that you need to fill with positive energy! The Yoni Egg helps with that.

Can the Yoni Egg be dangerous or toxic?

Yoni Eggs are perfectly safe if used properly, with the aid of a practitioner, and cleaned properly. In the thousands of years women have been using them, no one has ever gotten sick from using one.

What other crystals do you use regularly?

I keep Black Tourmaline near the computer to cleanse any EMFs in my space, and I use this stone for grounding as well as during new moon and full moon rituals. I also use Rose Quartz in bathing rituals.

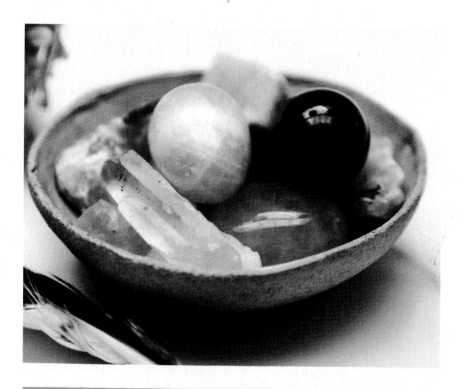

Now that you've met my friends and colleagues who are changing the game when it comes to all things crystal, let's move on to which crystals to pick when consulting the sun, moon, and stars based on your personal astrology. And oh yeah, why it energetically matters which finger you choose when you *put a ring on it.*

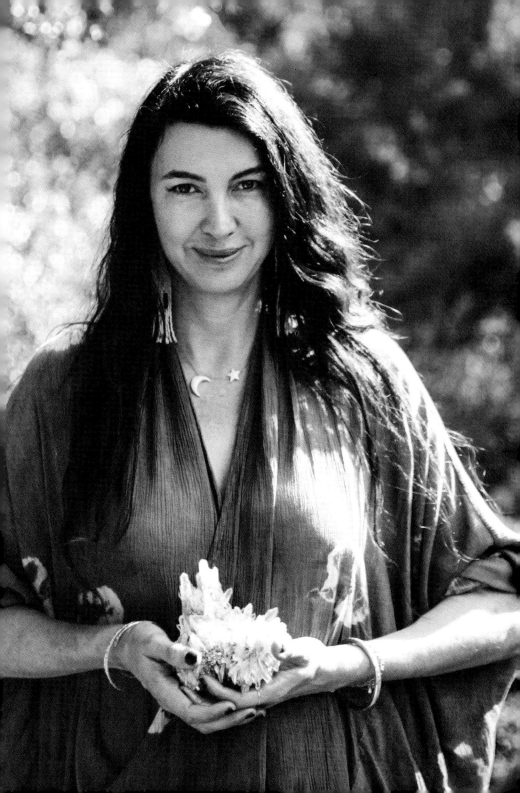

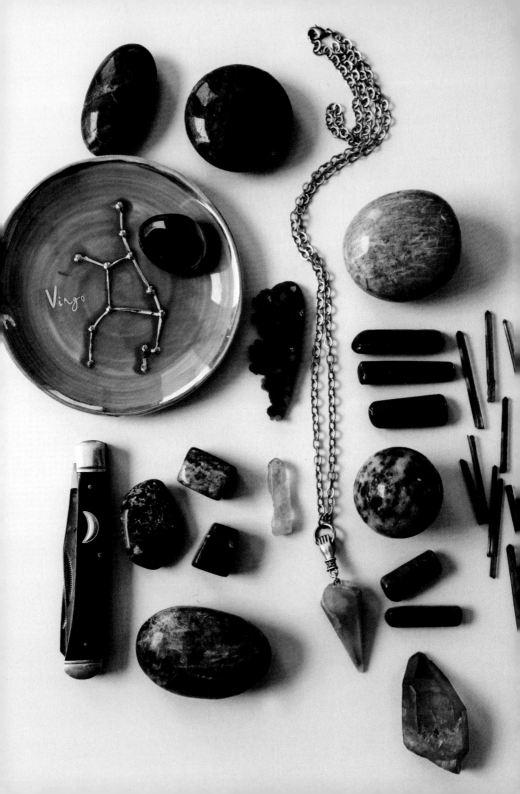

6

CRYSTALS AND THE ZODIAC

We have calcium in our bones, iron in our veins, carbon in
our souls, and nitrogen in our brains. 93 percent stardust,
with souls made of flames, we are all just stars that have
people names.

–NIKITA GILL

LET ME BE CLEAR: I am *not* an astrologist. However, in my line of
work, astrology comes up a lot. For example, I'll be at a dinner party
where an astrologer friend pulls up my chart (on an app) to explain, in
astrological terms, why I have *the feels* that day. This inevitably leads
to a conversation about why my Saturn is running extra laps around
its pastel-hued rings (i.e., why I need to learn certain lessons around
workload and boundaries). My response is that there is a crystal to help.
Eureka! Crystals can be perfect companions to a celestial reading. Each
type of stone out there resonates with a particular astrological sign,
and it's useful to know what crystals work best for you depending on
your sign.

WHAT'S YOUR SIGN?
AND WHY DOES IT MATTER?

Why is your sign important? (Aside from its use as a cheap pickup line!) Zodiac signs are based on the belief that people have strong, predetermined personalities and traits, depending on the conditions of their birth, including when they were born and the positions of celestial bodies at the time they were born. Astrology involves the study of personality types and their relationships to one another, and this can help you in your personal and professional life by allowing you to better understand yourself and how you react in different situations, how others perceive you, and how to work with people of other personality types.

Astrology employs a tool called a "natal chart" or "birth chart," which is a map of where all the planets were at the time of your birth. By using the exact time, date, and place of your birth, we can use a natal chart to determine how the positioning of the planets influences the very core of who you are. It's a common misconception that you are *only* one of twelve astrological signs. Each of us is actually a celestial amalgam of the Zodiac signs, meaning that you're a unique combo of your sun sign (which is what the magazine horoscopes discuss), as well as your moon sign, rising sign, Venus sign, and much, much more. Your personal starry blend helps determine every aspect of who you are: what clothes you like to wear; what colors you gravitate toward; how you choose to work, live, play, and socialize; the people you choose to date; and how you communicate with others.

These are the important elements to pay attention to on your natal chart, which go beyond whether you are technically Virgo, Aries, or Pisces, with info on how they relate to your crystal practice:

YOUR SUN SIGN

Your sun sign is determined by the day and month of your birth. It represents your Zodiac personality: your basic nature, your core traits, and who you are as a person when you're not consciously thinking about how you may be acting. Your sun sign explains why you like what you like and why you do things in a certain way.

YOUR MOON SIGN

Your moon sign is determined by the cycle of the moon at the time of your birth. Your moon sign represents your inner self and your emotional underbelly, the hidden side of who you are that you don't normally reveal to people. Have you ever had someone say to you in a stressful situation, "You're not acting like yourself. What's up?" This most likely means that your moon sign was coming out to play. If the moon can move the ocean and affect the tides, why wouldn't it also affect humans, who are roughly 70 percent water?

YOUR RISING/ASCENDANT SIGN

Your rising sign is determined by the Zodiac sign that was ascending on the eastern horizon the moment you were born. It represents the way others see you, and the first impressions that you give off. Upon meeting you, people will interact with your rising sign, and many people wear their ascendant sign as a kind of mask. Have you ever been perplexed by how others describe you? They are describing your rising sign, which may not align with the way you see yourself.

YOUR VENUS SIGN

Your Venus sign or love sign is determined by the position of the planet Venus at the time of your birth. Venus is your attraction factor, including how you attract monetary abundance, love, and any of the other things that you may want. Venus governs how you view relationships, what you want from a relationship, how you behave in a relationship, and the type of person you are attracted to. Please note: We're talking about who you are attracted to, *not* who you are actually compatible with.

CRYSTAL RX FOR YOUR STAR SIGN

Now that you have a basic handle on the birth chart, and how astrology is about more than just your "sign," I'd like to introduce you to some of the crystal healing methods I prescribe for my clients, depending on what's going on in their celestial worlds.

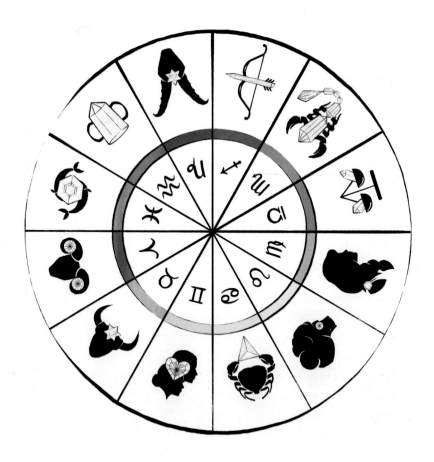

1. ***Karmic Kismet:*** There are six pairings of opposing signs in the Karmic Wheel of Astrology, aka the 7–7 Zodiac. If you count the signs on the wheel, your "karmic opposite" will be seven signs away from your sun sign. Opposites attract on the Zodiac, and opposing signs have complementary characteristics. You know those people in your life who you feel magnetically attracted to, even though they push your buttons and you are polar opposites? These oil-and-water pairings actually make us stronger, more balanced and complete. You two are "karmic medicine" for each other. With crystals, it works the same way. I often prescribe crystals that represent a client's karmic opposite on the astrology wheel in order to address the challenges they are working on.

THE 7-7 MIX 'N' MATCH

1. Aries-Libra
2. Taurus-Scorpio
3. Gemini-Sagittarius
4. Cancer-Capricorn
5. Leo-Aquarius
6. Virgo-Pisces

As an example, let's take the karmically opposite pairing of Virgo, sign of the Healer, and Pisces, sign of the Dreamer. Virgos are known to be grounded and organized, while Pisces are creative and emotionally expressive. Let's say a Virgo and a Pisces are working on a project together at work. If the Virgo is feeling stuck and the anxiety of a deadline is looming, she can embrace the energy of Pisces by working with Ocean Jasper to calm her overactive thoughts and do some out-of-the-box problem solving. On the flip side, fluid and dreamy Pisces may need to embrace Virgo's energy and write a team meeting agenda for the upcoming project with the help of some Amazonite.

2. ***Sun Meet Moon:*** We want to be full spectrum gem-bosses, right? This means we need to look at our personal polarity, aka the opposing sides of who we are. Each of us has a sun side and a moon side, depending on the situation. I also like to refer to these two opposing sides as "sparkle" and "shadow." And there are crystals we can use to address these polarities. When shamans work with someone's moon side, we are taking a look at that person's dark side, or shadow, whereas a person's sun side, or sparkle, represents the opposite.

    As an example, let's imagine someone whose sun sign is Sagittarius and whose moon sign is Aries. The sparkly side of this Sag is that she is an extroverted truth-seeker who loves to travel. This person's shadowy Aries moon side makes snap decisions with a hot temper to boot. Imagine that this globetrotting Sag is traveling in a foreign country, and decides she wants to hop on a train to get from point A to point B. Only when she arrives at the train station, there are no more seats available, because Sag didn't book ahead. Sag's moon in Aries shows up and throws a tantrum for the ticket booth attendant. To ground our wanderlust-y Sag, let's prescribe Black Obsidian with a side of Sodalite to keep her calm during travel and keep that hot-tongued mouth on ice.

3. ***Spin the Zodiac Wheel:*** Below are all the zodiac signs with a list of the stones and crystals that resonate for each. You can use this list to formulate your own Crystal Rx. Flex your intuitive muscle and pick from the suggested list of crystals for your sign, based on your gut and what you've read about each crystal elsewhere in the book.

HOUSE OF ARIES

The Ram

Birthdate: March 21–April 20

Featured Crystals: Agate, Amethyst, Blood Agate, Bloodstone, Carnelian, Citrine, Diamond, Fire Agate, Green Calcite, Iron Pyrite, Kunzite, Pink Tourmaline, Red Jasper, Red Tiger's Eye, Ruby, Watermelon Tourmaline

Planetary Positioning + Elemental Ally: Mars + Fire

Calling Cards: action-oriented, assertive, courageous, change, independence, fiery, passionate, overcoming obstacles, self-confidence, sexual, strong, vitality

Celestial Power Colors: Red and Orange

Chakra Association: 3rd/Solar Plexus

HOUSE OF TAURUS

The Bull

Birthdate: April 21–May 20

Featured Crystals: Amber, Emerald, Jade, Malachite, Pink Mangano Calcite, Rainbow Moonstone, Rose Quartz, Sapphire

Planetary Positioning + Elemental Ally: Venus + Earth

Calling Cards: patience, persistence, loyal, reliable, stable, lovers of beauty

Celestial Power Colors: Green or pink

Chakra Association: 4th/Heart

HOUSE OF GEMINI

The Twins

Birthdate: May 22–June 21

Featured Crystals: Agate, Citrine, Labradorite, Opal, Yellow Jasper

Planetary Positioning + Elemental Ally: Mercury + Air

Calling Cards: adaptability, good communication skills, intelligent, versatility, negotiations, positive, uplifting

Celestial Power Colors: Yellow

Chakra Association: 5th/Throat

HOUSE OF CANCER

The Crab

Birthdates: June 22–July 22

Featured Crystals: Citrine, Emerald, Lemurian Quartz, Milky Quartz, Moonstone, Opalite, Pearl, Selenite

Planetary Positioning + Elemental Ally: Moon + Water

Calling Cards: sensitivity, kindness, nurturer, home and family, children and animals, fertility, protection, secretive, go-to confidante, emotional security, sexuality, magical, highly intuitive

Celestial Power Colors: Silver

Chakra Association: 6th/Third Eye

HOUSE OF LEO

The Lioness

Birthdate: July 23–August 23

Featured Crystals: Amber, Black Onyx, Carnelian, Fire Opal, Fire Lemurian, Gold, Iron Pyrite, Red Spinel, Ruby, Sunstone

Planetary Positioning + Elemental Ally: Sun + Fire

Calling Cards: ambitious, courage, nobility, self-confidence, power, pride, prosperous, protector, talented, show(wo)man

Celestial Power Colors: Gold, Royal Blue, Purple, and Red

Chakra Association: 7th/Crown

HOUSE OF VIRGO

The Maiden

Birthdate: August 24–Sept 22

Featured Crystals: Amazonite, Chrysocolla, Green Aventurine, Green Calcite, Jade, Peridot, Peacock Ore, Serpentine, Snow Quartz

Planetary Positioning + Elemental Ally: Mercury + Earth

Calling Cards: Perfectionist, organization, methodical, task-oriented, list makers, efficient, detail oriented, dependable, love routine

Celestial Power Colors: Green, Blue, Lilac

Chakra Association: 5th/Throat

HOUSE OF LIBRA

The Scales

Birthdate: August 23–October 23

Featured Crystals: Amethyst, Blue Lace Agate, Blue Sapphire, Chrysocolla, Lapis Lazuli, Rainbow Opal, Tourmaline

Planetary Positioning + Elemental Ally: Venus + Air

Calling Cards: harmony, ability to see both sides, balanced, peacemakers, strong sense of justice

Celestial Power Colors: Light Blue and Indigo

Chakra Association: 4th/Heart

HOUSE OF SCORPIO

The Scorpion

Birthdate: October 24–November 22

Featured Crystals: Black Opal, Garnet, Hematite, Mahogany Obsidian, Malachite, Red Spinel, Rose Quartz, Titanium Quartz

Planetary Positioning + Elemental Ally: Pluto + Water

Calling Cards: intensity, transformation, birth and death cycles, psychic awareness

Celestial Power Colors: Red, Crimson, Black, Indigo, Purple, Burgundy

Chakra Association: 2nd/Sacral

HOUSE OF SAGITTARIUS

The Archer

Birthdate: November 23–December 21

Featured Crystals: Amethyst, Aragonite, Aqua Aura Quartz, Clear Quartz, Goldstone, Peacock Ore, Topaz, Turquoise

Planetary Positioning + Elemental Ally: Jupiter + Fire

Calling Cards: expansive, creativity, optimism, truth seeker, clear vision, world traveler, exploratory, flexible

Celestial Power Colors: Purple, Dark Blue, Yellow, Scarlet, Light Brown

Chakra Association: 3rd/Solar Plexus

HOUSE OF CAPRICORN

The Goat

Birthdate: December 22–January 20

Featured Crystals: Black Onyx, Garnet, Green Aventurine, Hematite, Jet, Mexican Tiger's Eye, Petrified Wood, Sardonyx, Smoky Quartz, Tiger's Eye

Planetary Positioning + Elemental Ally: Saturn + Earth

Calling Cards: cautious, task-master, self-discipline, loyalty, ambitious, persistent, traditional, prudent

Celestial Power Colors: Brown, Green, Gray, Indigo

Chakra Association: 1st/Root

HOUSE OF AQUARIUS

The Water Bearer

Birthdate: January 21–February 18

Crystals: Amethyst, Angelite, Celestite, Garnet, Sodalite, Sugilite, Titanium Aura Quartz, Turquoise

Planetary Positioning + Elemental Ally: Uranus + Air

Calling Cards: idealistic, independent, humanitarian, unique, inventive

Celestial Power Colors: Dark Purple, Blue

Chakra Association: 1st/Root

HOUSE OF PISCES

The Fish

Birthdate: February 19–March 20

Crystals: Amethyst, Aquamarine, Bloodstone, Fluorite, Girasol, Ocean Jasper, Pink Kunzite, Sugelite, Watermelon Tourmaline

Planetary Positioning + Elemental Ally: Neptune and Jupiter + Water

Calling Cards: intuitive, empathetic, fluid, adaptable, creative

Celestial Power Colors: White, Mauve, Light Green, Silver, Blue

Chakra Association: 3rd/Solar Plexus

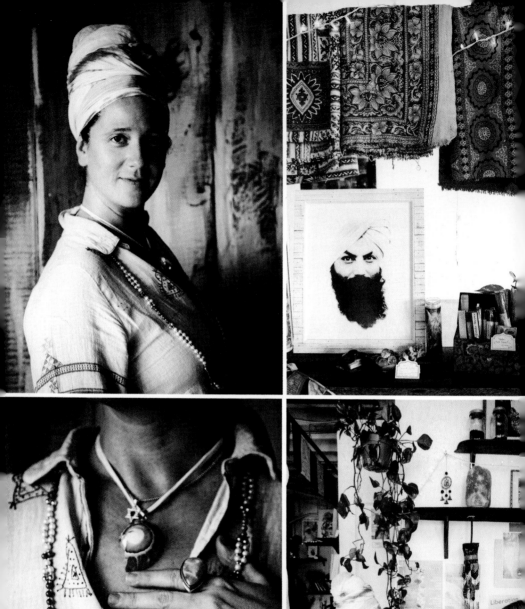
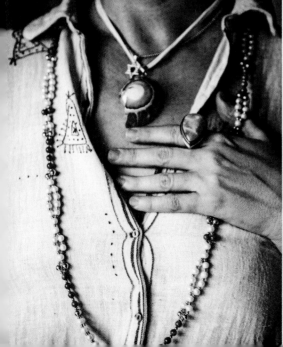
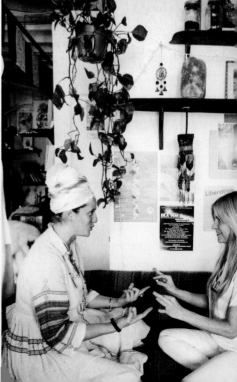

Interview with Guru Jagat, Founder of RA MA Institute for Applied Yogic Science and Technology

I LIVE JUST DOWN THE STREET from the RA MA Institute in Venice, California, which means I get to call Guru Jagat and the Aquarian Women's Leadership Council my neighbors. Guru Jagat, RA MA's Founder, is the youngest senior Kundalini yoga teacher in the world and the face of the new Kundalini movement. Kundalini yoga is a blend of Bhakti yoga (the yogic practice of devotion and chanting), Raja yoga (the practice of meditation/mental and physical control), and Shakti yoga, (for the expression of power and energy). And the RA MA Institute is a gathering place for those who want to learn how to use Kundalini yoga and meditation to chemically release, strengthen, and activate their genetic code, while igniting the energy centers of the body, mind, and spirit. Guru Jagat has studio locations in LA, New York City, and Mallorca, and she's a complete force of nature—plus, she's funny, wise, and super humble.

When did you get into crystals?

I've been into crystals since I was a child, as they were part of my upbringing. It was a family affair. Growing up, my mom's friends were all Vedic astrologers and Reiki masters. My brother turned our kitchen into a temple and later on became a Hare Krishna. We hosted drum ceremonies on our land regularly as well. We were highly spiritual vegans living in rural West Virginia in the 1980s; nobody else in my grade school had crystals or was eating a broiled tofu sandwich at the lunch table.

When did Kundalini yoga come into your life?

I was looking for a teacher; I didn't realize at the time that was what I was looking for, but looking back, that's what I needed. I had moved to New York City in my early twenties and had tried the party scene, and that wasn't the right fit for me. I knew there was something beyond the eat, sleep, work, watch TV, have sex, and die matrix. I attended a "weird" yoga class right after 9/11, where the teacher was doing something called *Kundalini* and she wore a cool turban. Literally, within 20 seconds of being in the Kundalini class, I felt like I was home. I started studying with Yogi Bhajan at his ashram, and the rest is history.

How do astrology and crystals play into your yoga practice?

I want to be clear, I am not a Vedic astrologer—however, I do use the foundations of Vedic gem technology as an activator in my practice. (Vedic astrology, also sometimes called *jyotish* in Sanskrit, translates to "science of light." It's a mathematically based form of astrology describing the planetary patterns at the time of our birth. The Vedic tradition is distinctly different from what we think of as Western astrology, as it uses the sidereal zodiac, which is based on the fixed, observable positions of the constellations as we see them in the sky. Western astrology, in contrast, uses what is called the tropical zodiac. The tropical zodiac is based on the changeable position of the sun, rather than on the fixed, observable positions of the constellations.) I believe that we can activate certain planetary aspects by wearing certain gems on certain fingers. My teacher, Yogi Bhajan, says that our fingers are "antennae" for planetary activation. These are the "Planetary Rings" that he believes you should wear on certain fingers to activate certain things:

- JUPITER FINGER (pointer): Yellow Sapphire
- SATURN FINGER (middle): Blue Sapphire, Hessonite, Cat's Eye, or Diamond
- SUN FINGER (ring): Ruby or Coral
- MERCURY FINGER (pinky): Emerald or Pearl

PLEASE NOTE: *Rings should only be worn on the middle or Saturn finger for very specific reasons and by spiritual masters. Please consult a professional before engaging in this practice.*

If you were a crystal, which one would you be?

Tibetan Clear Quartz, because of my connection to Tibet. There's something really incredible and ancient about it.

Since you now know how to put on your crystal best from head to toe, from the inside out, and from here to the cosmos, it's time to go on a little road trip. Trade in your high heels for hiking boots, as we are about to get dirty in the very best of ways. I am taking you off-off-road to meet some of my favorite people in the most faraway places.

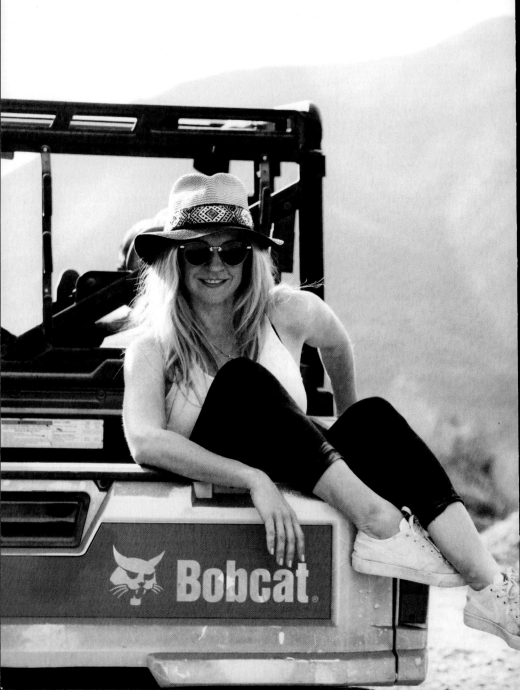

7

LET'S GO EXPLORING!

Be lionhearted. Be nerdy as f***. Stay sexy. Remain
intelligent. Be courageous. But, above all, embrace
the sh*t out of your insanity.

—ERIN VAN VUREN

WHAT'S THE MOST COMMON REQUEST I GET from editors and clients alike, aside from what must-have crystal they should have in their life? It's "Can I travel with you? Take me with you!" In this chapter, I want to do the next best thing by sharing some of the most gem-tastic adventures I have been on, from the high mountains of the Andes to the cavernous crystal caves of California that are practically in my own backyard. Get ready for a snapshot of how I learn, connect, work, and play with gem lovers from all over the world. Who do I hang out with? Where do we go? Finding new crystals to add to my collection through my travels is always so exciting, and every stone has a story.

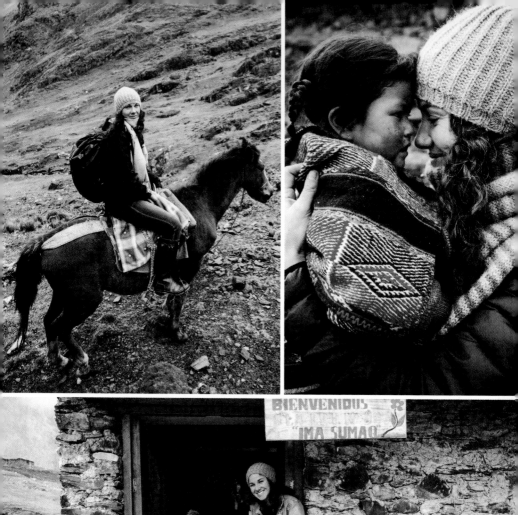
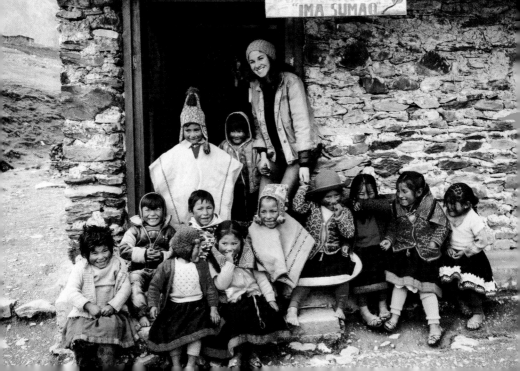

Interview with Hannah Rae Porst, Founder of Willka Yachay

HANNAH HAS BEEN LIVING IN PERU FOR ALMOST A DECADE, collaborating with and learning about the wisdom of the Andes from the Q'ero shamans. Hannah is an incredible person, a total badass, and the founder of a nonprofit that supports the indigenous people of Peru.

How did you start Willka Yachay? And what is the organization's goal?

I was twenty years old when I first heard of the Q'ero people and felt in my heart that I needed to travel to their mountain home to meet them. Once I did, I fell in love with them, their culture, and the mountains. I spent time researching the intersection of indigenous culture and global development, and during a community dinner one night, I asked village parents how I could thank them for their hospitality. There was initial talk about soccer shoes, but what they really needed, they told me, was a school. So in our early years of working together, we built and opened preschools, elementary schools, a high school, and a school for adults. Today, Willka Yachay's goal is to help indigenous communities thrive in the modern world. We are empowering the Q'ero people of Peru to elevate their standard of living, guide their community toward sustainable modernity, and preserve their cultural identity.

Could you describe your training as a shaman?

Over the past several years, I have been formally apprenticing with the Q'ero medicine men and women. One of my teachers, Cipriana, is one hundred years old and has never left her mountain home. I have been blessed and initiated with centuries-old healing stones and crystals, transmitting energy cultivated through the ages. I am grateful for what the Q'ero people have taught me about how to love and revere our natural world.

Can you tell us about your work with crystals?

During my seventh year working with the Q'ero, I was riding a horse up at 16,000 feet at the base of Waman Lipa, the most sacred mountain in the Q'ero tradition. A voice told me to get off my horse and that a heart-shaped crystal would be waiting for me. I jumped off my horse, walked ten steps and looked down in amazement to see a heart-shaped crystal. I used this stone to start my *mesa*, my Andean healing bundle.

EXPLORING THE ORIGINS OF STONE MEDICINE IN PERU'S SACRED VALLEY

A big part of my training has involved studying Peruvian shamanism with the Q'ero in Peru, who are modern-day descendants of the Incas and pioneers of stone medicine. I want to take you on an adventure through Peru's Sacred Valley, where the Q'ero live between 16,000 feet and the Amazon Basin. They have settled along select points of this area, at various altitudes, where they engage in activities like farming, tending animals, weaving, and selling goods. This area is wild, raw, and magnificent, and the mountains cradle you at every turn. I recently traveled to the Sacred Valley to document one of the origins of ancient stone medicine with photographer Amy Dickerson and Hannah Rae Porst, founder of the Peruvian NGO Willka Yachay, which is an organization dedicated to supporting all members of the Q'ero community and fostering sustainable development and a strong intercultural connection between the Q'ero and the outside world.

We began in the city of Cusco in southeastern Peru, and journeyed into the mountains, called the *apu*, which have long been revered as gods and spirits at the center of ancient Andean spirituality. This unforgettable pilgrimage pushed me to my physical limits, as we tackled steep climbs, navigated narrow mountain passes, and dealt with incredibly cold weather at dizzying altitudes.

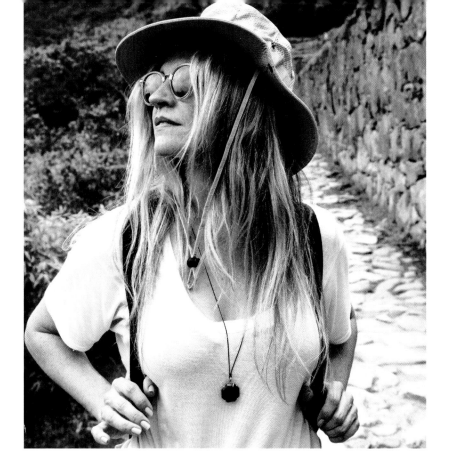

PASS THE SALT: THE MARAS SALT FLATS

One of our first stops was a tiny town in the Sacred Valley called Maras (located at 11,890 feet), known for its tiered salt ponds, which have been in use since pre-Incan times. Since Incan times, the salt harvested from these ponds has been freely available to all members of the Maras community. Halite is the mineral name for the substance we commonly know as salt, and its metaphysical properties are vast, including:

- Attracting abundance and manifesting desires
- Promoting healing, physical well-being, and longevity
- Providing spiritual protection and purification

- Providing insights on life, death, and spiritual rebirth
- Balancing emotions and tapping into altered states like dreaming and meditation
- Preventing spiritual "decay" (Many religions and spiritual modalities sprinkle salt, or create circles, lines, or piles of it, for this purpose.)

THE CITY SURROUNDED BY QUARTZ: OLLANTAYTAMBO

The next stop on our journey was the town of Ollantaytambo (9,160 feet), an Incan archaeological site located along the Willkamayu, or Sacred River, in the Sacred Valley. Formerly the home of Incan nobility, Ollantaytambo is now a popular tourist destination and starting point for the four-day, three-night hike along the Inca Trail to Machu Picchu. There is a great shopping market in the middle of the town with a plethora of handwoven goods for sale. But the most impressive part of shopping is looking up at the town's ancient stone backdrop: pre-Incan terraces and megaliths that are made of mostly Quartz crystal. The stone isn't local, but was dragged from the other side of the valley. How the ancient builders moved mountain-size stones that great distance remains a mystery today, although many archaeologists have theories.

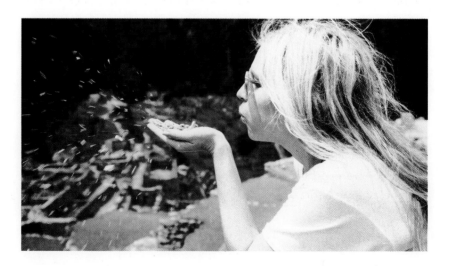

THE OG CRYSTAL CITY: MACHU PICCHU

Following Ollantaytambo, we boarded a train to Machu Picchu (8,040 feet), arriving after nightfall in the town of Aguas Calientes, which sits at its base. Machu Picchu, which means "old mountain" or "old peak," is a fifteenth-century Incan citadel that was built as an estate for the Incan emperor Pachacuti Inca Yupanqui. And it, too, is primarily made of Quartz. Its primary buildings are the Intihuatana ("Hitching Post of the Sun"), the Temple of the Sun, and the Room of the Three Windows. The four sides of the Intihuatana represent the four compass directions (north, south, east, and west) and the Medicine Wheel in shamanism, and the structure was used for astronomical observations and ritual ceremonies. Only the priests and the Inca were allowed to enter the Temple of the Sun, which was used as a solar observatory and a place for animal sacrifices. In the Room of Three Windows, the three remaining windows (there were originally five) each represent a part of the world: Ukhu Pacha (the Lower World), Hanaq Pacha (the Upper World), and Kay Pacha (the Middle World, or Present Time on Earth).

Machu Picchu is not just a mysterious architectural feat with breathtaking views of Peru's mountains. It also happens to be an energy vortex. Vortexes are high-energy sites that can be found all over the world. Other well-known vortexes include Sedona, Stonehenge, and the Great Pyramids of Giza. The energy of vortexes can't be detected by the naked eye, but we can measure their effects with divination methods, and with tools like a pendulum or a magnetometer. Vortexes often have high-vibe stones, which store information and harness energy, placed on the land by Mother Nature (Sedona) or designed by man (Stonehenge, Machu Picchu). Most vortexes have a heavy concentration of Limestone, Quartz, and Magnetite. Why did the ancients build these ancient structures on top of vortexes using stones and crystals? They believed that they could use them to create, transmit, and channel energy—sort of like acupuncture needles that worked with the earth's energy. Travelers visit well-known energy vortexes for a variety of reasons, from contemplating the meaning of life to increasing their physical wellness to looking for their next big business idea—and many claim to have found these things at vortexes, Machu Picchu included.

PLAYING DRESS-UP WITH SEÑORA VALENTINA!

One of my favorite moments on the trip was being carefully and lovingly dressed by one of the elders of the community, Señora Valentina, who happened to be the village fashion plate. I felt a bit like a five-year-old girl trying on my mom's high heels! Valentina pulled out her favorite pieces and advised me on all the key items. My favorite piece was a *pollera*, a *very* heavy wool square dancing–esque skirt decorated with embroidery, beading, rickrack, and sequins. Valentina told me that on an average day, Q'ero women wear three or four skirts at a time! Not only for style, but for warmth. I don't have an exact weight on the skirts, but it is a full-time job wearing one. The finishing touch was when Valentina added a colorful 4-inch-wide woven belt, tied even tighter than the skirt (which was tight!) to exaggerate my shape. How these badass mountain women can herd llamas, do their daily chores, or even breathe in these skirts is beyond me.

Señora Valentina and her family members Señora Maria and Señor Jose Luis also wanted to show me how to hand-dye baby alpaca fibers, which are used in the beautiful textiles and weavings of the Q'ero. They put on their Sunday best and treated our dyeing lesson as a ceremony. We sat next to the rushing river and used insects, dried herbs, flowers, natural indigo, and crystals to color the fibers. The fibers were first spun into yarn, then dipped in the dye, then cooled and dried and handed over to the women to make the colors come to life in their beautiful weavings. Designs are specific to family groups or tribes (*ayllu*), as textiles are representative of specific communities and their cultural heritage. Additional decoration in the form of tassels, brocade, feathers, and beads made of precious metals or shells is then added to the weavings.

WEAVING THE STORIES OF THEIR LIVES

Q'ero women have been using looms to weave for centuries. A *wichuna*, or llama bone pick, is used to weave images of animals, lakes, rivers, plants, spirits and other sacred symbols that bring meaning in everyday life through the vibrantly dyed alpaca fibers. Women weave most textiles and garments, though men do make *chullos,* ear-flapped Andean hats. A Q'ero woman's knowledge of motifs and her skill at weaving fine cloth increases not only her status in the community, but also her ability to provide for her family. The Q'ero women weave the stories of their lives and their ancestors into their textiles. Storytelling through weaving is one of the most important ways the Q'ero people preserve their cultural traditions.

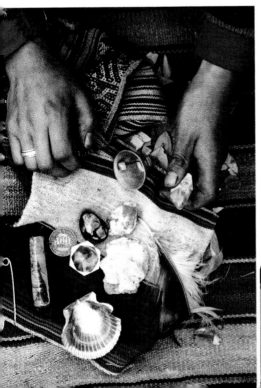
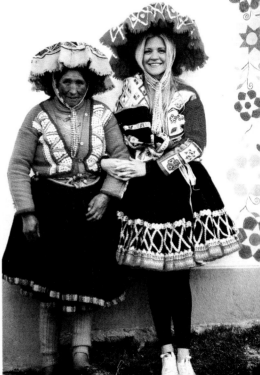

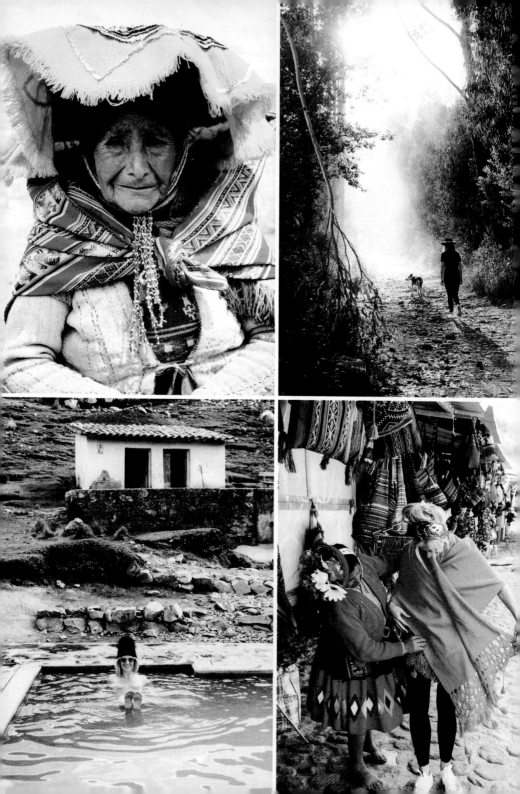

Textiles are an integral part of Q'ero life from birth to death. When babies are born, they are wrapped in the traditional *mestana* cloth, which, as they enter into adulthood, becomes their personal medicine bag, or *mesa*. When death comes, Q'ero people wrap the deceased in their finest cloth for burial. Clothing has always been a symbol and indicator in Incan society of a person's wealth, status, and region and family they come from.

SHAMAN CENTRAL: QOCHAMOQO

Our next stop, the most dangerous and exciting part of our adventure, began in the village of Qochamoqo (14,500 feet), which has the highest concentration of resident shamans of any of the fourteen high-mountain villages that are part of the Cordillera de Vilcanota mountain range.

To get there, we had to drive for eight hours southeast of Cusco with our guide Santos and horse-wrangler Raymundo on windy mountain back roads through small villages, and down dirt roads, with wild dogs often running alongside the car and old women in vibrant outfits waving from their doorways.

The president of Qochamoqo Village, Alejandro Ordoñez, was there to greet us at the start of our trek up the Apu Waman Lipa, along with eight horses and a few community members to escort us up the mountain. To ascend Waman Lipa, you must travel on horseback, wearing a backpack that holds, along with your other supplies, a small, portable oxygen tank because of the altitude. The guides led our horses on a two-hour-long climb, at 45-degree inclines. We navigated skinny rocky trails as herds of llama and alpaca frolicked around us. We had to be prepared for whatever weather conditions the mountain would throw at us, from clear blue skies to torrential downpour. The journey was treacherous, but I felt completely safe climbing with our guides, who know the mountain like the back of their hand.

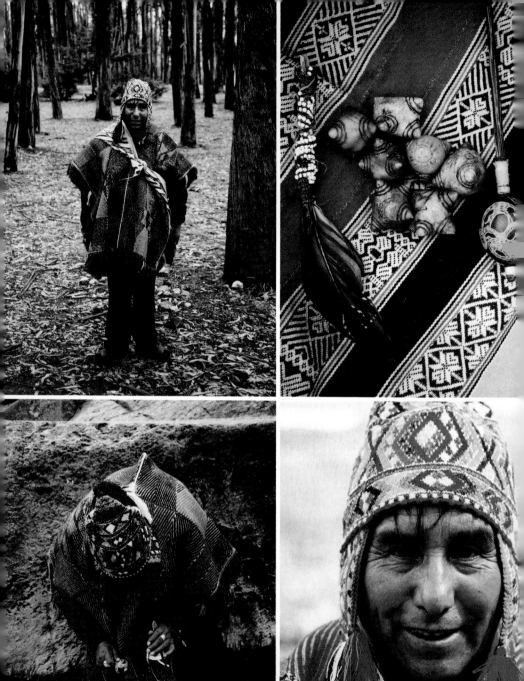

Interview with Don Augustine, Third-Generation Q'ero Shaman

WHILE VISITING PERU'S SACRED VALLEY, I was lucky enough to spend time with third-generation Q'ero Shaman Don Augustine. He is an *altomisyoq*, which means "wisdom keeper," and he is the highest level of Andean ritualist, one who is traditionally known to directly converse with the *apu*, or "mountain spirits," on behalf of the people.

How were you chosen as a shaman in your tribe?

First, the Apu Waman Lipa sent dreams to my father, who was also a shaman, that I was to be a shaman. Next, my father went to have my coca leaves read to confirm that this was true. Once it was confirmed, I was able to begin my training. I then received the first initiation rite from my father.

Where did you get the stones in your mesa?

Many of the stones are from my father, grandfather, and older generations. A spirit came to my father to tell him I was allowed to use the stones to heal people. My father was given permission by the spirits to pass the stones to me. The other stones were received as gifts from the mountains or through *karpays* (shamanic rites of initiation).

How many years have you been a shaman and who do you work with?

I am fifty-eight years old and have been a practicing shaman for thirty-two years. I started my initiation rites when I was sixteen years old. When I first started to work, it was with the Q'ero people, and now I also work with the foreigners that come to visit Cusco. I would also like to come to North America and work.

What energies do you work with?

Apu Waman Lipa is my medicine. I received my first initiation at Apu Waman Lipa and feel most connected with the energies of this place.

If you were a crystal, which crystal would you be?

Clear Quartz

Upon reaching the summit at 16,000 feet, the spectacular sky-blue Scissor Lake comes into view when you look down a deep ravine. I truly felt like I was on another planet as we dismounted our horses at the summit and took a stretch and a group photo. For the next leg of our journey, the descent, we had to hike back down the mountain on foot, because the incline is too steep to ride on horseback, which took about an hour. The guides lovingly slapped our horses on the ass to let them know it was time to go, and they tore off down the mountain. It became dark, cold, and rainy as our hike progressed, and then finally Qocham-oqo Village, with its picturesque stone and straw-thatched houses peppered across the hill, reappeared out of the mist.

We were invited to stay overnight in the 150-year-old family home of our guide Santos and his father, Shaman Don Augustine (see page 241). We were as out of pocket and off the grid as could be, with no indoor heating, plumbing, electricity, or WiFi. We slept on a bed of llama skins and wool blankets at night, and what was lacking in modern-day creature comforts was more than made up for by the warmth of our hosts.

I had long heard my shaman teachers talk about the importance of respecting and worshipping the *apu*, but I didn't fully appreciate what they meant until this trip. Coming face-to-face with the mountains at those altitudes and in extreme weather conditions with nowhere to hide was so humbling. And I was often in awe of the Q'ero people, who are so tough. I would stand there freezing in my parka and boots, next to the smiling Q'ero who don't wear closed-toed shoes (only a flip-flop-like sandal to cover the sole of the foot over rocky terrain) or heavy jackets because their bodies have acclimatized to the weather.

THE ULTIMATE JOURNEY: SHAMAN SCHOOL

Ten years into my crystal journey, after spending time as a student at the Four Winds, a school of energy medicine; receiving my training as an Usui Reiki master; continuing intuitive study with my teachers; and founding Style Rituals, the universe asked me to step even deeper into the healing world. Stephen Feely, a mentor and former teacher from the Four Winds, approached me to say that said he was founding a Peruvian-based school called Pampamesayok Shaman School (*pampamesayok* meaning "earth keeper" in Quechua) in his home state of Tennessee, and he wanted me to be his co-teacher. I was honored, but also intimidated. Crystal healing is only one aspect of shamanism. Did I really know enough about shamanism, its lineage, and everything that goes along with it to accept this position? As we say in shamanism, Stephen was *holding space* for me to step into a role as teacher. He said I was already teaching in my private sessions, and he knew I could do it. So I said yes!

WHAT DO WE TEACH AT SHAMAN SCHOOL?

Our teachings focus on Peruvian-based Incan shamanism; however, we sprinkle Nordic, Chinese, Siberian, and Mexican shamanic traditions into our curriculum. The curriculum we teach is Shamanism 101, and it's the perfect place to start if you are interested in learning about shamanism for self-healing or want to become a shamanic practitioner. We teach The Medicine Wheel, which is the foundational teachings of shamanism (more on that later), and we also teach practical ways to incorporate these ancient wisdom practices into your daily life by combining aspects of psychology, neuroscience, quantum physics, cultural anthropology, mysticism, and a bit of alchemy. Our curriculum is also largely based on what is taught at the Four Winds, and we teach it with the permission and blessings of Four Winds founder Alberto Villoldo.

WHAT IS THE MEDICINE WHEEL?

Stepping up as a shaman in your community means you agree to become a *pampamesayok*, or "earth keeper." As a *pampamesayok*, you take on the responsibility of caring for the land and its inhabitants to the best of your ability with your gifts and skill set. In each of the four directional classes, different components of our being are examined on a physical, emotional, mental, and spiritual/energetic level. Each direction represents aspects from each of the following categories:

1. Stages of life (birth, youth, adult, death)
2. Seasons of the year (spring, summer, fall, winter)
3. Elements of nature (fire, air, water, earth)
4. Animal archetypes (animals vary per shamanic lineage; in the Peruvian tradition we speak about the serpent, jaguar, hummingbird, and eagle/condor)
5. Sacred herbs (sage, cedar, sweet grass, tobacco),
6. Through "directional" storytelling on a symbolic level, ancient teachings and hands-on healing practicum that accompany each direction, we are able to guide and empower our students into a personal journey of transformation.

WHO COMES TO CLASS?

Shaman School is open to anyone who feels called to attend. In our classes, we see a lot of healthcare professionals who are looking to add a new skill set to their current practice, whether they're psychologists, acupuncturists, massage therapists, nurses, hospice workers, counselors, meditation and yoga teachers, or Reiki practitioners. Other people we see? Those in community leadership roles, executives, public relations and marketing directors, ministers, human resource consultants, and motivational speakers. And then there are the wild cards, like firefighters, rocket scientists, and fashion stylists (ahem!). Our classes are typically around 80 percent female, but come on guys! The door is wide-open.

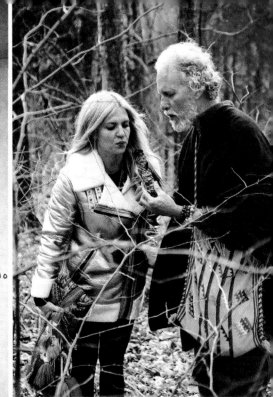

'elcome ♡ to
Shaman School

are luminous beings on
a journey to the STARS.
+ you have to experience
nfinity to understand." — Don Antonio

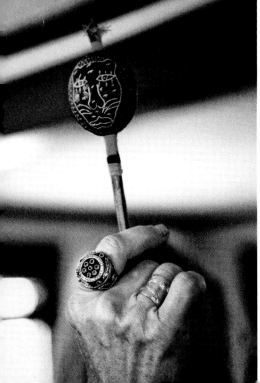

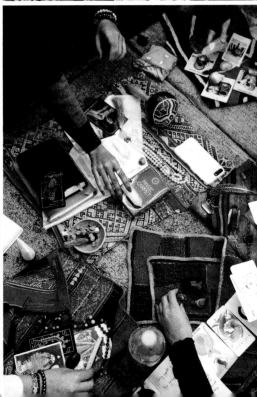

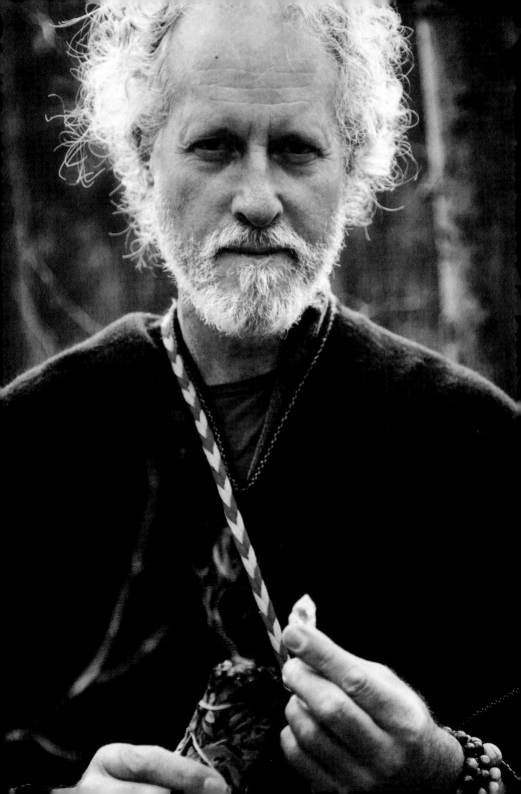

Interview with Stephen Feely, BSA, RP, HLB, Founder of Pampamesayok Shaman School

STEPHEN AND I ARE LIKE PEAS AND CARROTS when we get together to teach: Stephen speaks with great poetic wisdom and thirty years of shamanic experience, and I bring the beauty and sparkle through ceremony and ritual, and by making sure we have a killer altar decorated to perfection. Stephen is a certified energy medicine practitioner, Usui Reiki master and senior faculty member at the Four Winds. Besides his energetically inclined accolades, he is also a writer, father, community leader, biodynamic farmer, environmental educator, and one of the wisest and most interesting people I know. He is most known for sharing his deep connection to the healing forces of nature.

When did you first get into crystals?

I started collecting stones as a child, and many of these became the stones that are in my shaman medicine bag today. I have been playing with stones forever. In middle school, I had a geology teacher who took us out rock-hunting and really opened my eyes as she talked about the spirit of rocks and their properties. This experience was really formative, and I started associating rocks with a sense of place and a profound knowing of the dynamic qualities of the earth. I grew up farming with my family, and I knew that when I touched rocks and placed them in certain places, it meant something. My whole life, my interest in crystals has been led by a sense of play, wonderment, and creativity!

How do you use crystals in your shamanic work?

I use crystals in a session to create a safe and inviting space for the heaviness that may be in a client's Luminous Energy Field. It's like the light of the crystal is "mulching" the energetic heaviness and turning it back into light. That is what shamans do—we honor the heaviness, and we love it back to a high vibration so that it can become light. My crystals are like a support team that I can use to activate a healing intention. I think of them as a bridge between earth and sky, and this is the pathway I travel when I journey to support a client in his or her healing or intention.

What was it like for you to study with the Q'ero?

Humbling. These medicine men and women live in a space of never having forgotten why we are here and who we are as human beings. It's like the innocence we're all born with has never been extinguished in these extraordinary men and women and their beautiful children. Studying with them has allowed me to discover a new fuel within myself, allowing me to claim a kind of second innocence. The Q'ero are very wise, yet they should never be put on a pedestal. They are some of the most authentic human beings I have ever met. And therein lies their magic.

What is the most rewarding part of your work?

Watching people get back in touch with how beautiful their souls really are, once they let go of all the stories that tell them otherwise, and as they return to love and claim an empowered path to walk forward into their destiny.

What else do we need to know about crystals?

No matter how many crystals we humans collect during our time on this planet, they will all eventually end up back in the earth. We are only borrowing them for a brief visit, and then the earth will take back what was borrowed. Our crystals choose us, knowing that we need their medicine to get back in touch with what it is to be human.

If you were a crystal, which one would you be?

Amethyst, because it changes through time. For example, recently I watched a particular Amethyst on my farm change from deep purple to a cloudy white. Then all these fuzzy, tiny crystals started forming on the outside of it. I started wiping off the crystal fuzz, aka baby crystal dust, and putting it into several beds of soil on my farm that were ready to be planted. The places where I added the dust, the plants grew bigger, stronger, and more flavorful. This particular Amethyst crystal then went back to being purple again. Amethyst is the most dynamic crystal I have ever seen, and it is its own playground of wisdom and transformation.

GOING ON A CRYSTAL DIG

I recently went with a bunch of my rock hound friends to dig for gems at the Pala Chief Mine, in Pala, California. Pala Chief is one of the oldest gem mines in San Diego County, and it's one of the only historic mines still being actively worked in the hunt for American gemstones. It's a freestyle dig, so you bring your own tools: bucket, shovel, hand rake, pry bars, rubber gloves, and toothbrush. All you have to do to get in on the crystal madness is to book an appointment through their website and pay a fee. We were on the hunt for gems the mine is best known for: Aquamarine, Garnet, Kunzite, Morganite, and Quartz.

Crystal Digging at Pala Chief Mine, Step by Step

1. Put on sunscreen, sun hat, and your hot pink gardening gloves!
2. Fill your bucket with a pile of dirt, rocks, and gems to sift through.
3. Carry the bucket to your designated station and dump everything over the $\frac{1}{4}$-inch mesh screens to sift through what you have.
4. Submerge your screen in water.
5. Pick out the larger rocks first, then grab your toothbrush. Gently scrub each stone with the toothbrush to see what treasures were covered by dirt.
6. Take your screen out of the water and select the stones you want to keep.

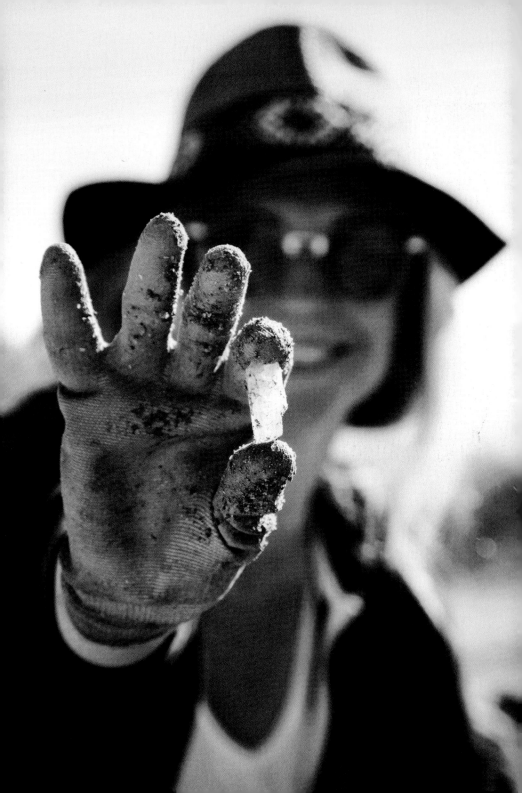

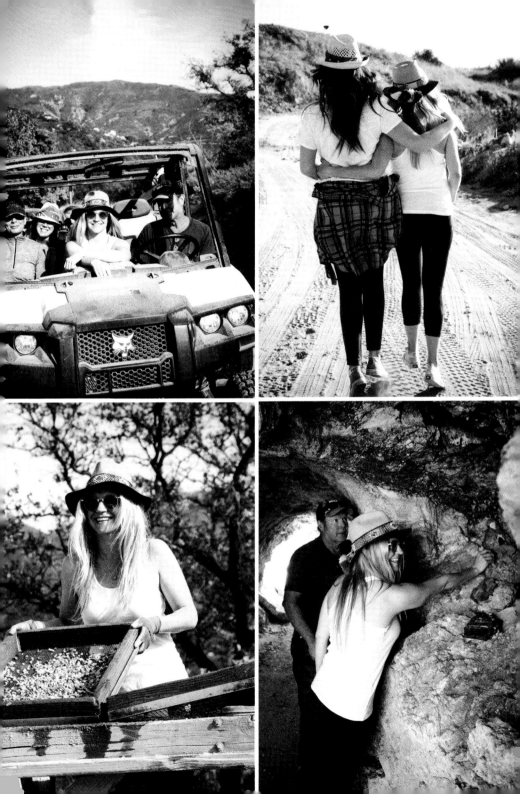

TAKE IT TO THE BANK!

Most of the miners at Pala Chief have been doing this for years, and are trained and certified in various specialties. On this most recent trip, we got to hang out with Steve Carter, who is an expert in drilling and blasting (he knows a lot about explosives!). Steve offered to take us on a personal tour of the mine, and needless to say, we were all fighting for shotgun in his golf cart! As Steve whisked us through the canyon hills, he gave us the rundown on how the Pala Chief Mine got started. It was originally owned by J. P. Morgan and George Frederick Kunz, an American mineralogist and former vice president and buyer for Tiffany and Co. Along with being a money man, J. P. Morgan was also a notable gemstone collector and was responsible for funding some of the world's greatest gemstone collections, which can be seen in museums today. In 1911, J. P. Morgan's contribution to the gemstone world was acknowledged when Kunz named a newly found gem, Morganite, after the financier. They also discovered Kunzite, named of course for Kunz.

We ended our day at Pala Chief with plenty of gems in our pockets, but also super dirty and dusty—sort of like emerging from the Mojave after Burning Man. Caution: DO NOT wear anything you care about to either event.

THE TUSCON GEM SHOW: GEM SHOPPING IN THE WILD WEST!

The Tucson Gem Show is the oldest, largest, and sparkliest in the world. It takes place every year in late January or early February, and this year I headed out there to see gem distributors and colleagues, and to visit one of my mentors, Brian Cook, who is one of the top experts on ethical gem mining in the world. I also had a lengthy shopping list from private clients with me! The experience is always incredible: Running around Tucson, literally hugging Smart car–size gems, and sitting in a carved Rose Quartz bathtub were a couple of the highlights from this year.

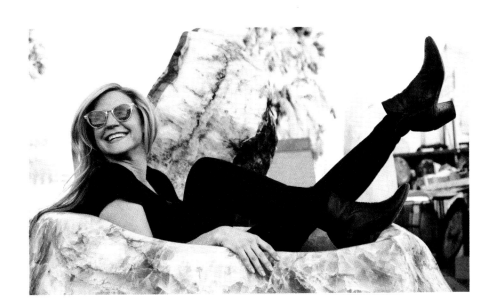

There are two main tents at the show: the American Gem Trade Association (AGTA) tent, and the Jewelers Circular Keystone (JCK) tent. The tents of these two big crystal organizations house all the high-end pieces at the Tucson show, and you need to be in the gem business or have an all-access press pass to get in. Once inside, you get to interact with everyone from Smithsonian gem geeks to technologists promoting the newest lasers for gem cutting. In addition to what's going on in the tents, there is also a symposium given by experts from around the world. Lectures and interactive experiences start with a sage energy clearing in the morning, followed by sessions that cover jewelry retailing, cutting and mounting gems, technological advancements, education and professional development, ethical practices, and Oscars-style design awards.

Tips for Navigating the Wild West of Crystal Shopping

- Bring your tax ID! Purchasers must have a retail business and proof of the business with resale certificate.
- Crystals are heavy AF! Bring a TSA-approved carry-on or a collapsible grandma-style grocery cart. If you get really crazy with

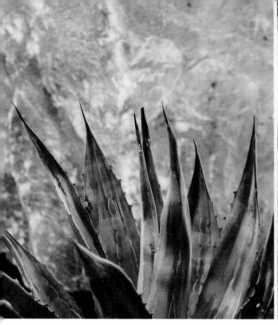
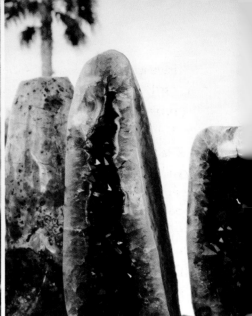

your purchases, or buy the "big one," the vendor or your friendly neighborhood UPS will help you get them home safely.

- What to wear? I came in with a blow-out and left with a dusty, disheveled top-knot. You're going to be in and out of the hot Arizona sun all day, so wear sunscreen, a hat, and some sh*t-kickers you don't mind getting dusty and that you can stand in all day.

- Drink plenty of water. The combination of desert weather and energetic vibes from the crystals will leave you sucked dry and with a nasty high-vibe hangover the following morning if you don't.

- The official gem show starts at the end of January, but serious buyers and deal-hounds are already lurking around Tucson in mid- to late January, hoping to be the first to score.

- How do I speak the purchasing lingo?

  NET: The purchaser pays full the price marked on the label.

  KEYSTONE: 50% off the price marked.

  DOUBLE KEYSTONE: 75% off the price marked. (That's like hitting the big one at the craps table!)

  WHOLESALE: 50% off the price marked. The purchaser must

have a retail business and have proof of the business with resale certificate. All wholesalers require resale licenses.

INTERLAGOS: These letters correspond to the numbers 1234567890. A mineral priced "TAG" = $378.

- There is no standard pricing system at the gem show, so when you first arrive in a dealer's room or tent, look for any of the terms mentioned above. These will indicate the pricing plan used by the dealer. If there is no indication of pricing, ask the dealer how the minerals are priced to avoid confusion during checkout. P.S. Yes, you can barter!

- Cash is king! It's a rookie mistake to think you can use plastic in the parking lot, which is where all the vendors who aren't in the AGTA or JCK buildings with the expensive gems set up shop. There are literally parking lots, hotel lobbies, and sidewalks with makeshift crystal tent cities throughout Tucson during the show. The entire town turns into a gem market! You don't want to find yourself pleading with a Brazilian dealer to let you send him some PayPal love for a piece you just can't leave behind (like I did recently!). Bring cash!

A combination of following my intuition, a nomadic way of life, and my wanderlust nature has led me to continuously jump down one mystical rabbit hole after another. I am super blessed to be greeted on the other side by diverse people and their deeply rooted spiritual traditions and rituals everywhere I go. I am grateful to be welcomed into so many "tribes" who have helped fuel my love, education, and exploration of all things sparkly so that I, in turn, may share my knowledge and experiences with you. My crystal adventures will continue to be an integral part of my work as a healer because it is the one aspect of my work that unifies everything I have ever done, and continues to ignite my curiosity and inspire me.

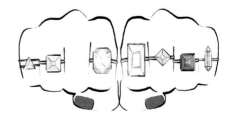

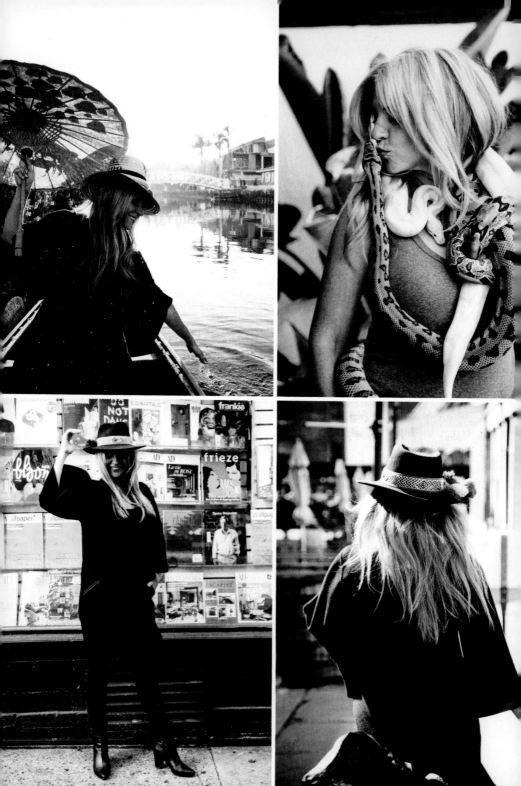

THE CRYSTAL LIFE

I HAVE ALWAYS BEEN ACUTELY AWARE of the power and strength that lies in the exquisite. With an intuitive eye for trends, I began my journey in the world of fashion, and eighteen years of style-centric pursuits allowed me to wear many hats—first as a designer, stylist, and brand consultant and now as a shaman who "prescribes" crystal statement jewelery as a conduit for healing, views a closet as a snapshot of someone's psyche, and storyboards with tarot cards and gems to reveal a person's past, present, and future. The ancient art of crystal healing is finding its way into the modern world, and I am honored to be a steward for crystal medicine and to give this subject a much-needed facelift, new design sensibility, and an understandable language that works for the modern day. Crystals are also becoming big business and it's important to have a palatable dialogue that aligns the age-old and the cutting edge, explaining how mysticism meets science, and how Eastern modalities can walk hand in hand into the sunset with Western medicine. If I had to coin a name for this trend board, I would call it #AncientFuture . . . although I hope it never goes out of style. I feel a great responsibility to share the knowledge I have gained with my clients, and now my readers. I hope that this book will inspire you to embrace crystals and bring them into your daily lives, so that you can experience the power of their healing, their energy, their inspiration and their beauty for yourself.

Muah! Colleen

ACKNOWLEDGMENTS

GRATITUDES: My thank-yous could go on and on, as I truly believe everyone you come in contact with shows up as a teacher to you in some form or another. I want to thank some very special people who have been my guiding light, my compass, my confidants, my voices of reason, my medicine, and my calm within the middle of a mystical sh*tstorm so many moons ago.

To the women who helped to put my best visual foot forward: Eva Gajzer, founder of Office of Oneness, who has been a dear friend and my business strategist since Style Rituals was born. Judith van den Hoek illustrated all the crystal-y fashion sketches in this book and on the website. My book photographer, Amy Dickerson, you followed me to sixteen thousand feet and back with no questions asked, a smile on your face, and always up for anything . . . I couldn't have told this story without you. Jamie Young, my manager, you provide so much wisdom when it comes to navigating every rabbit hole we jump down. Jessica Sindler, my editor at HarperCollins, for always helping me to remember to keep a beginner's mind in all I do. My assistant, Sabrina Crockett, for helping me keep my sh*t together.

To the women in the fashion and beauty community who first RSVP'd "yes" to the notion that sage and stilettos can party together: Ruby Warrington, founder of the Numinous, and Chioma Nnadi, fashion director of Vogue.com. I owe a deep thank-you to the editorial world for supporting my business, giving me a soapbox to stand on, and teaching me how to become a writer. A special thank-you to GOOP, *Vogue*, *Time*, Well+Good, the Numinous, and L'Oréal.

To the people in my spiritual community, for being my guiding light on an esoteric road less traveled. My teachers at the Four Winds: Dr. Alberto Villoldo, Marcela Lobos, Stephen Feely, Peter Bonaker, Ruby Parker, Dean Taraborelli, Jim Dewell, Julie Hannon, and Elise Kost. My intuitive mentors Asa Hoffman, Marisa Pouw, Betsey Bergstrom, and Reiki Master Raemonica Patterson. My crystal mentors "Shey-Shey," Brian Cook, Kirby Seid, and Master Jeffrey Yuen.

My family: Mom, Dad, Caitlin, Carrie, Tootsie, Aunt Sissy, Grandma McCann, and the rest of the McCann Clan.

My loved ones, allyu, and colleagues: Thank you for being my guinea pigs when I said, "Look what I can do with crystals!"; housing me in your spare bedrooms when I was on my mystical walkabout; supporting me through the weird and wild; drying my tears and holding my hand on the hard days; making me laugh; connecting me to other amazing people along the way; and adventuring with me to faraway places. Priestess "Ace" Cartter Evans, Kelly Conroy, Christopher Germain, Christina Carathanassis, Kara Kiensicki, Katherine Killeffer, Katherine Mapother, Brian Bowman, Lauren Hack, Vanessa Ungaro, Danielle Donahue, Derek Reynolds, John-Miller Monzon, Annie Ehrmann, Lindsey Fuerur, Tiffany Jackson, Lee Schwalb, Ashley Brothers, Taryn Davis, Tanaaz Chubb, Joelle Arondoski Michaeloff, Christine Schuster, Joel Douek, Satnam Ramgotra, Hekesha, Kin, Astrid, and my O.G. adventure buddy Nicole Thomas.

My clients, you have been my greatest teachers, helping guide me on what to tell the world about stone medicine and so much more in this book.

Those who offered their insight for this book: Q'ero peoples of Peru, President Alejandro Ordoñez and the people of Qochamoqo Village, Andi Scarbrough, Zoe Taylor-Crane, Dr. Mona Dinari, Kirby Seid, Brian, Kendra and Quendi Cook, Guru Jagat, Brook Harvey-Taylor, Adina Mills, Anjanette Sinesio, Carolyn Ford, Einstein, Paul Martinez, Consuelo Casarotto, Don Augustine, Hannah Rae Porst, John Murphy,

Joyanne "Joy" Prebyl, Justina Blakeney, Madeleine Murphy, Mona Dinari, Señor Jose Luis, Señora Maria, Señora Valentina, Shey Shey, Shiva Rose, Shaman Stephen Feely, Katherine Wildt, Kristen LaLumiere, Cam Ochs, Lindsay Marias, Sally England, Jamie Bechtold, Londin Angel Winters, Helena Krodel, David Wegweiser, Kerrilynn Pamer, Cind DiPrima, Heather Tierney, Santos and Raymundo, Walter, Tobias and Alysha, Justin Guizar, Ashley Abbot, Rockstar Crystal, Mystic Journey, House of Intuition, Spellbound Sky, Earthen Warrior, Putchipuu, Pound Pendulum, and of course my Spirit Guides.

Thank you all for being the token magic that I carry with me everywhere I roam.

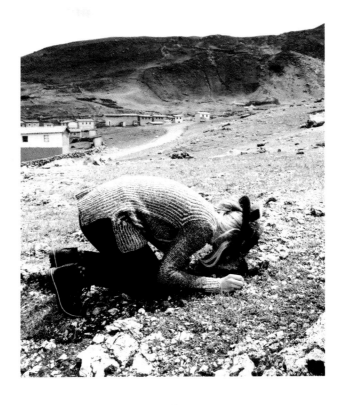

CREDITS

Cover photograph and interior images by Amy Dickerson

All illustrations by Judith van den Hoek

Color wheel on pages 52–53 courtesy of *The Seven Secrets of Crystal Talismans: How to Use Their Power for Attraction, Protection & Transformation* by Henry M. Mason © 2008 Llewellyn Worldwide. Used with permission.

Photographs on pages 60–77 and 110–43 by Wayne Stambler and Sara Essex Bradley

Prop styling on jacket by Rose Thicket-Justina and Trevor Freel

ABOUT THE AUTHOR

COLLEEN MCCANN is a certified Shamanic Energy Practitioner who was a fashion stylist in a past life. She has traveled the world researching crystal traditions and conducting crystal readings, as well as space clearing and balancing, shamanic healing, and intuitive business coaching sessions. She is a regular columnist for Time.com, and her work has been featured on GOOP and in *Vogue*, the *New York Times*, *W, Vanity Fair,* and Refinery29. She lives in New York and Los Angeles. Her website is www.stylerituals.com.

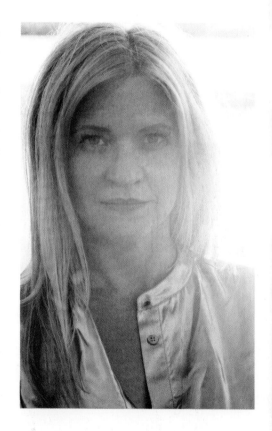